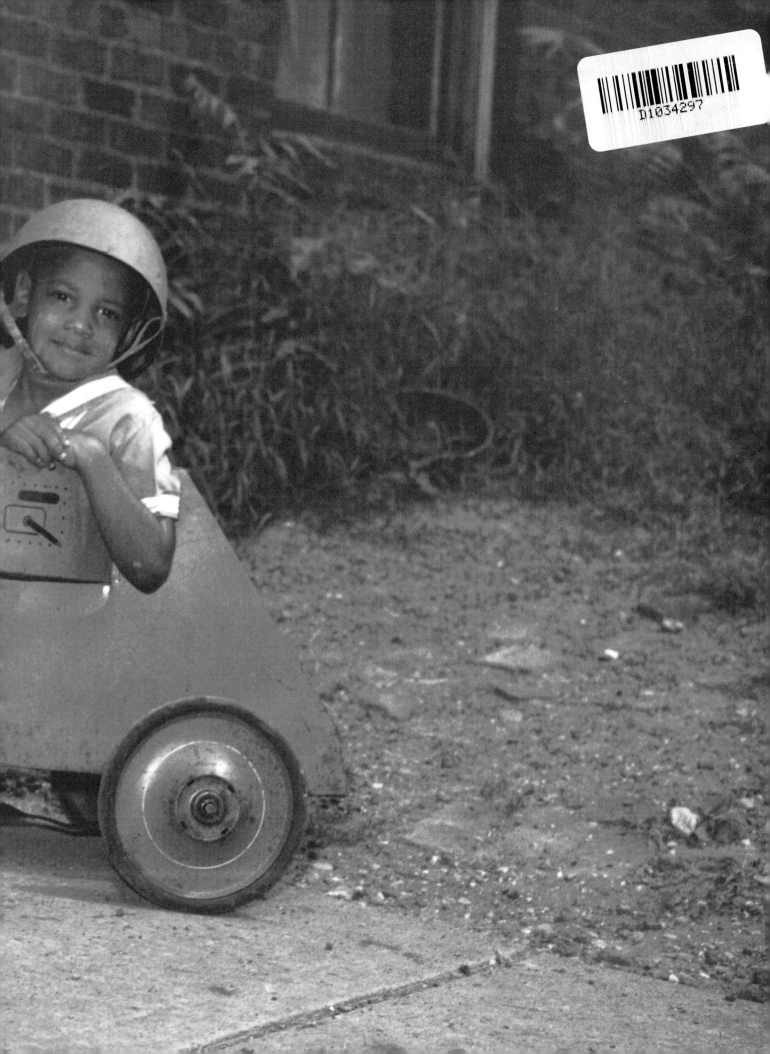

Wee Warriors
and
Playtime Patriots

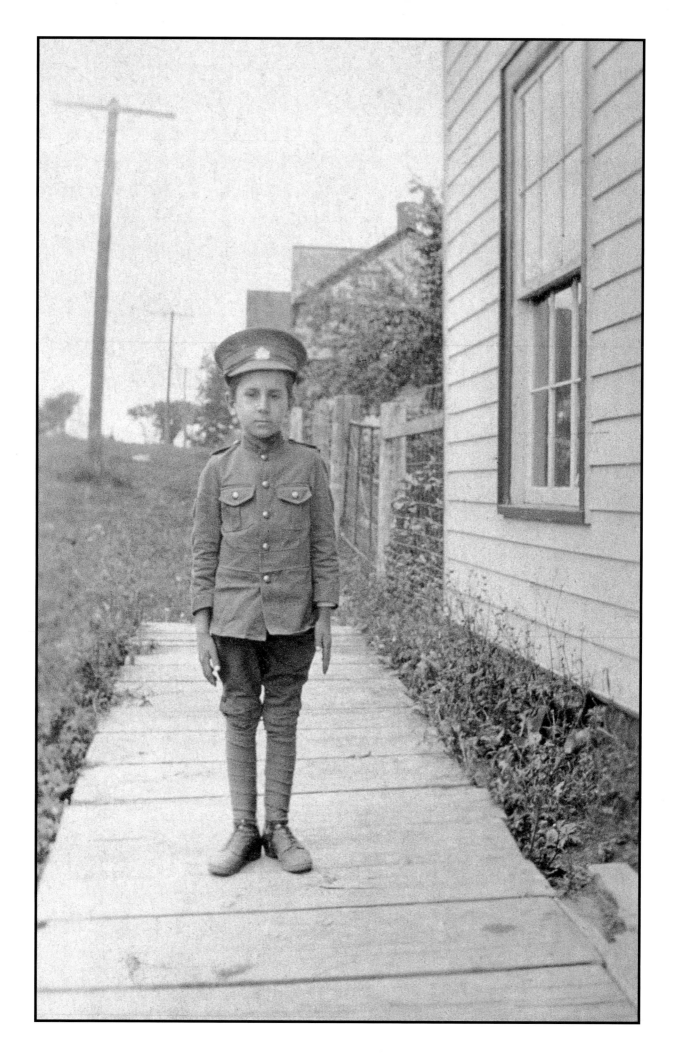

Wee Warriors and Playtime Patriots

*Children's Military Regalia:
Civil War through the Vietnam Era*

Nancy Griffith

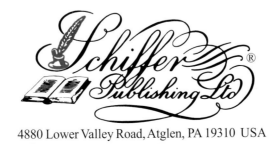

4880 Lower Valley Road, Atglen, PA 19310 USA

Designed by "Sue" and Lydia Inglett Spears
Type set in Geometr Hv BT/Korinna BT

Sears Roebuck Catalog pages are used by permission of Sears Roebuck & Company, Archives Public Relations and Communications Department, 3333 Beverly Road, Hoffman Estates, Illinois 61079; (847) 286-2500.

Montgomery Ward Catalog pages are used by permission of the University of Wyoming American Heritage Center, P.O. Box 3924, Laramie, Wyoming 82071-3924; Michael Devine, director; Daniel Davis, photographic archivist; (307) 766-4114.

Captions, portions, and adaptations from "The Young Cavaliers: An Introduction to Boy's Swords," reprinted and used by permission of *Man at Arms Magazine,* 1525 Old Louisquisset Pike, Lincoln, Rhode Island 02865-4524; Stuart C. Mowbray, editor; Joseph Puleo, technical editor; (401) 726-8011.

Adaptations and captions from *Zouaves: The First and the Bravest* by Michael McAfee, 1991, Thomas Publications Gettysburg, Pennsylvania, and are used by permission.

Technical drawings of "Terminology of the Sword and Scabbard" and "Nomenclature of the Hilt" are adapted from *The American Sword 1775-1945* by Harold Peterson, 1977 (4th printing), Ray Rilings Arms Books Company, Philadelphia, Pennsylvania, and are used by permission of the publisher.

Campbell Soup® and The Campbell Kids® are trademarks of the Campbell Soup Company, Campbell Place, Camden, New Jersey.

"Over There!" Words and music by George M. Cohan (1917).
"Anchors Aweigh," ©1907 Robbins Music Corporation, New York, New York; words by Capt. Alfred H. Miles, USN; revised lyrics by George D. Lottman; music by Charles A. Zimmerman, USN+.
Back end sheet from the Franklin D. Roosevelt Presidential Library archives.
All other photos are used by permission or are the property of the author.

ISBN: 0-7643-1181-6
Printed in China

Published by Schiffer Publishing Ltd.
4880 Lower Valley Road
Atglen, PA 19310
Phone: (610) 593-1777; Fax: (610) 593-2002
E-mail: Schifferbk@aol.com
Please visit our web site catalog at **www.SCHIFFERBOOKS.COM**
We are always looking for people to write books on new and related subjects. If you have an idea for a book please contact us at the above address.

This book may be purchased from the publisher.
Include $3.95 for shipping.
Please try your bookstore first.
You may write for a free catalog.

In Europe, Schiffer books are distributed by
Bushwood Books
6 Marksbury Ave.
Kew Gardens
Surrey TW9 4JF England
Phone: 44 (0) 20 8392-8585; Fax: 44 (0) 20 8392-9876
E-mail: Bushwd@aol.com
Free postage in the U.K., Europe; air mail at cost.

Dedication

For my friends and family.
Here and there, now and then.

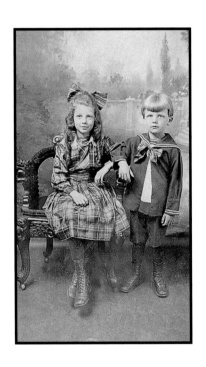 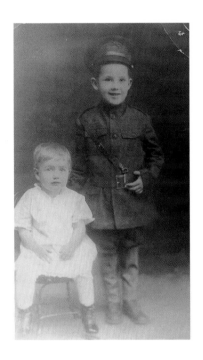

Contents

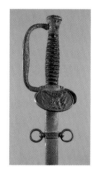

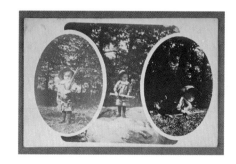

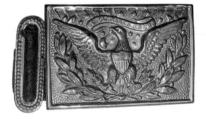

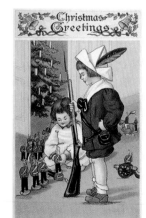

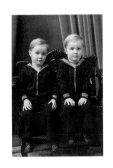

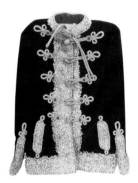
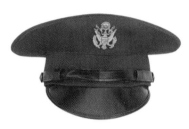
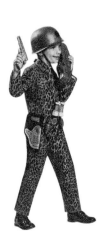

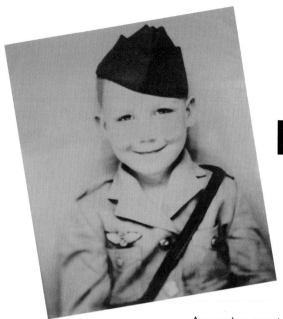

Foreword

As senior curator of a major American museum, I have come in contact with many military collections in my career. I have viewed items from every war or conflict this country has ever been involved in. After a while, all of the items tend to become redundant. There are just so many flight jackets, visor hats, helmets, guns, and swords that one person can see.

However, individual collectors still find it fascinating that I make my living sorting through copious amounts of personal memorabilia as well as government-issue items that for one reason or other American servicemen finally give to the museum for posterity's sake.

What happens is that my tastes and those of other professional curators gravitate to the unknown as well as rare—rare in the sense that most individuals never run into items from these unusual classes.

It is at this crossroad where the sublime to us (rare to most) no longer possesses the unique qualities I referred to above. To garner my interest is to pique it. The information you will read about in this reference book certainly piqued that interest.

One thing universal in every one of the wars and conflicts noted above was that children were left behind when their fathers and mothers went off to war. Psychologically, this was indeed a burden upon parents who were left behind not only to raise their children in single-parent households but also to explain to these young people exactly why their parents had gone off to war and just what they were doing while they were away.

It is with somewhat mixed emotions that I relate that information. My own father was a professional military patriot. He was gone on campaigns before I was born as well as afterward.

It certainly was difficult for my mother to raise her brood by herself. It was equally hard on my father to leave knowing this responsibility shifted solely to her shoulders.

Why did children dress up in the uniforms of their parents? It was to ease several pains. Pretending to be just like them offset the loneliness of not having a father or mother. To don a costume and play soldier or sailor was not only a way to pass the time but to feel as though their parents had not left them. And for "stay-behind parents," seeing their children in uniforms soothed a troublesome pain, the pain of separation from loved ones. Sending pictures of loved ones, especially children, was a much-desired present for parents who were so far away. Whether on the beaches of Normandy, Okinawa, and the like, the frozen tundra of Korea, or in the boonies of Vietnam, there was nothing like receiving pictures of children, their children who were growing so quickly. Imagine receiving pictures of children dressed just like they were.

There could be no greater joy.

This work chronicles the history of one aspect of military service—the costumes or uniforms children wore while their parents were away at war. It covers the United States Civil War period to the Vietnam era. These uniforms at first were custom made from whatever material the stay-behind parent might have had on hand, but business eventually took notice, and the next thing we have are companies that produced them for profit.

The author of this publication, Nancy Griffith, has the most extensive collection of children's militaria that I have ever personally seen. She has acquired examples of this genre from around the world. I invite you to read, look, and imagine all of those young people parading around, marching to and fro with just one thing in mind—to be like their moms or dads.

Robert R. Macon
Senior Curator/Deputy Director
National Museum of Naval Aviation

Preface

For as long as men have marched off to battle, little boys have stayed behind and played war. Even so, at the endless procession of antiques stores and flea markets that my husband and I frequent, I still get puzzled looks from busy vendors when I inquire about children's military dress.

Conversations usually go something like this: "Hi, I was wondering if you have anything in the way of children's military play uniforms or costumes? "I ask.

"Hmmm, children's military play uniforms or costumes?" vendors repeat, enunciating every syllable so deliberately that I can't tell if it's for their own benefit or mine. "You know, I don't think so." This is the cue for my husband, Steve, to head down the aisle to the next booth. "I didn't even know they made such a thing," they continue.

"OK, well, thanks anyway," I say politely as I turn to leave.

"But you know," vendors often add, "I think I know what you may be talking about." I stop, smile, and turn to hear what I know is coming next. "I think somewhere I still have a picture of me and my cousin. He was all dressed up in a little sailor's suit."

By now, I am looking around for my not-quite-so-patient husband who is halfway down the next aisle of booths. "Bring it next month!" I yell. Flipping a business card onto a table, I run to catch up with Steve, knowing in my heart that the promised picture will probably never materialize.

As a former collector of nothing, I had always felt my life was fulfilling enough without the endless clutter and anxiety of a "collection" of anything. Furthermore, my attraction to the military-collectibles arena was not a natural draw. I married in.

My personal decision to assemble a collection of anything was made the first time I saw a child-size version of an adult military uniform at a military-collectibles show. Suddenly, and without warning, the tiny uniform captured my imagination as it lay before me on the table. My mind raced with strategies for justifying the purchase. I was

consumed, knowing I just had to own it. Ten minutes after plunking down my money to buy it, I not only had decided I must have more—many more—but I also knew I was going to write the book.

While my obsession took on a life of its own, I was at times saddened when I ran across a hat or coat that was not in what I considered "collectible" condition. As I was quick to learn, children's clothing items and accoutrements are often well worn or damaged when they turn up. Many saw double duty with younger siblings, often succumbing to roughhousing and constant wear, or were just outgrown and discarded.

Never let it be said that this curious little slice of Americana and its international counterpart served up here has hard-and-fast rules. Many of the uniforms and accompanying accessories on the following pages were tailored to resemble the real thing, right down to the very last intricate detail. Happily, though, most are the product of clever conjecture by moms or grandmothers who put them together from whatever materials were on hand. Others were the creative brainchilds of manufacturers or chain stores bent on taking full advantage of upward swings in patriotism.

Nevertheless, regardless of origin, age, or condition, they are all, without exception, extraordinary and tell a story about us as a society and country. With a few exceptions, I offer here examples specifically designed for the childlike fantasy of soldiering.

Countless books have already chronicled the details of specific wars, so I won't attempt to repeat facts that can be found elsewhere. I have endeavored only to gather a group of related items and identify them roughly with the wartime period they represent. No excuses, no apologies. Descriptions of manufacturing detail are provided only when available or when pertinent to specific historical value.

That's my story, and I'm sticking to it.

Nancy Griffith

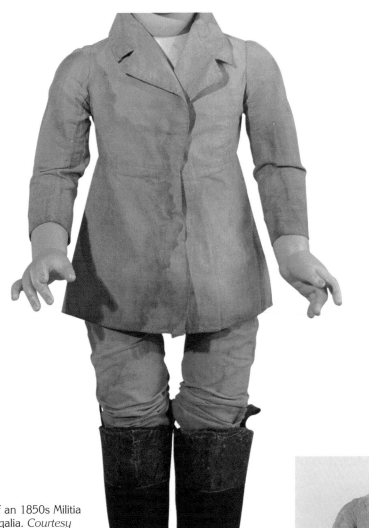

Below: A quarter-plate daguerreotype of an 1850s Militia officer and his son dressed in similar regalia. *Courtesy Rex Stark Americana.* Right: Suit made in 1846 by W.B. Turner for his three-year-old son, George, who wore it to accompany his father the day Mr. Turner enlisted to fight in the Mexican War. *Courtesy Jere Lee Hook Collection*

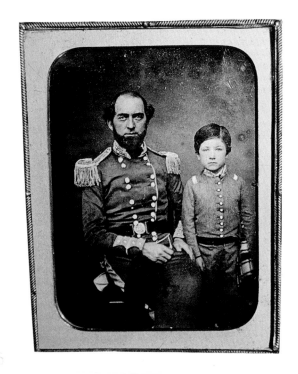

Acknowledgments

An effort such as this would not have been possible without the help of many people. I am humbled by the expressions of generosity and willingness to share artifacts, precious family memories, time, and knowledge and by the support, cooperation, and hard work I received. I thank you all from the bottom of my heart.

To Dennis Keesee and Michael J. Bremer, who provided so many wonderful photos and spent time patiently educating me on the nuances of their particular collecting interests. Stuart Mowbray and the staff of *Man at Arms Magazine*; Michael J. McAfee, Newburgh, New York; George Juno and Russ Pritchard; *North South Trader*; Michael Horestsky of Cocoa Curio Historical Militaria, Hershey, Pennsylvania; Steve Lister; Fred Jolly; Adel Gilmore; Charles Nohai; Jack Matthews; Thomas T. and Marie DiMartini Whittman; Tony Riley; Paul Wolfe and Martin Campbell, Riverwalk Antique Depot, Augusta, Georgia; Larry and Terri Stewart; Anthony Jessen; Bill Rasp; Herb Peck; Mike Constable; Jack and Debbie Buchert; The Naval Aviation Museum Foundation; Captain (Retired) Robert Rasmussen (director), Buddy Macon (senior curator/deputy director), Karen Thrower, Frank Matson, Sherri Shaw, Hill Goodspeed, and the library volunteers of the National Museum of Naval Aviation, Pensacola, Florida; Lauri Cosgrove, Charles and Nan Nash, and John Sexton of Stone Mountain Relics, Stone Mountain, Georgia; Clifford Orth; Everitt Bowles; Peter Coleman; John Conway; George Peterson; Walter Kanzler and Emily Caldwell Stewart; Chris and Jan Long; Joe Grosclose; Larry Baker; Jim Berry; Tom Kaleta Sr.; Gary Delscamp; Caryl Young; Rex Joyner; Franc Isla; Richard Peacher; Bill Curtis; Andrew Lipps; F. Pat Anthony; Bill Brooks; Steve Todd; Brooks Bush; John Bourke and Doug "Big Daddy" Hamilton of Philadelphia Street Antiques, Covington, Kentucky; Rex Stark Americana; Art Beltrone; Joe Riling; Vicki Cwiok, Sears Roebuck & Co., Photo Archives & Public Relations and Communications Departments; University of Wyoming American Heritage Center; the Jones family and their staff at Noble & Cooley Co., Granville, Massachusetts; Dennis Preisler of The History Factory; Manny and Andrew Scoulas (you started this!); Gailen David, my freshman-year head cheerleader; Fred Villarreal for building my show displays; Lon & Dawn Wassen for building my website; and Eric Olig Photography, Augusta, Georgia.

To Howard Hoffman and the officers of Forks of the Delaware Antique Weapons Association, officers of the Maryland Antique Arms Show (MACA) and the Tennessee Military Collectors Association (TMCA) for inviting me to their shows and graciously introducing me and my little-known area of collecting to their members and guests.

To Kathleen MacDonald and Debra Allen, my *camarades d'obsession* in our male-dominated hobby, your photos, friendship, and support are appreciated more than you know.

To dear friends and great hosts Bob and Danielle Chatt, Vintage Productions, Huntington Beach, California, for the extraordinary effort to gather some of the best material I have received.

To my fellow Schiffer authors Bob Baldwin, Nick Snider, Mick Prodger, Jon Maguire, and Warren Carroll for the advice, encouragement, support (and Glenlivet) I needed to take on this scary task.

The brilliance of my editor Leslie Nelson (who exorcised the demons), and art director Lydia Inglett Spears is acknowledged. My gracious thanks for putting up with my neurotic behavior and excuses, all while managing to turn this pile into something I can be proud of.

To my parents, Bob and Diane Guffin, who got excited and were proud of everything I shared when returning home from a trip, even when they didn't know what it was. My daughter, Lindsay, who helped me with the mundane tasks of information gathering, sorting, and labeling. To Lillian Guffin-Cross, Irene Pitchford and Hazel Bagby-Griffith.

To my wonderful husband, Steve Griffith, who shared his vast, unyielding knowledge; answered thousands of questions; and pointed me in the right direction to do the military research ("Is that what you wanted me to say, honey?"). Who said "no" to a lot of people, but never to me, and steadfastly had the wisdom never to say "I told you..." when I made costly mistakes in my collection. I love you dearly.

To David Foster for telling me, "You're not a writer."

Finally, to anyone else, individual or institution, I have inadvertently omitted, my thanks and apologies.

LITTLE PLAYERS. — PART I.

THE SOLDIERS.

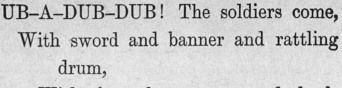

R UB–A–DUB–DUB! The soldiers come,
   With sword and banner and rattling
      drum,
      With feet that tramp and heels
      that stamp,
      They march in line from the nurs-
      ery camp.
   Oh, stiff and straight, with a rum-
      tiddy-um,
         The soldiers come!

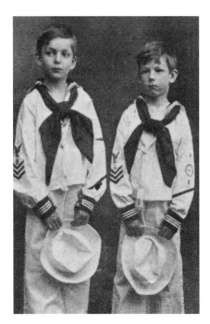

Part One: 1860-1940 An Introduction————

Dennis Keesee

Throughout history soldiers have battled, fought, and deservedly won admiration from countrymen. Great warriors were rewarded with land, money, and due fame. In a world before sports figures and media personalities took center stage, soldiers held highest honors. As young children, we were taught to imitate surroundings, including all basic life skills. Early we learned that good actions drew approval and support from our parents, and later from our peers.

During the 19th and first half of the 20th centuries when military personnel were elevated to hero status, children emulated soldiers' actions and daring feats through play. With sticks mindfully portraying swords and guns, playing war won the approval of adult onlookers who likewise were brought up respecting bravery and goodness.

Of all wars, the American Civil War shines as a passionately fought conflict that touched everyone in the country. It was not a war fought for land but for individual rights. Surprisingly, it was a conflict that saw thousands of young boys fight and die alongside older soldiers. Charles King of the 49th Pennsylvania infantry, at age 13, was mortally wounded at the battle of Antietam, Maryland, one of many youngsters who were sacrificed. For families that declined to allow their children to head off to war, the next best thing was to make military outfits for them, letting them play pretend soldier to their hearts' content. Most of the youngest recruits accepted by the military were used as musicians, and every boy in the land wanted a toy drum to play. With the patriot frenzy of the time, literally every child wore some sort of military coat or hat to school or play. Zouave-cut jackets were the fashion, and the blue in the North and butternut gray of the South were the colors of the day. When 15-year-old William Bircher marched off to war as drummer of the 2nd Minnesota, he noted the children watching the parade: "As we formed in line and marched down the main street towards the river, the sidewalks were everywhere crowded with people, with boys who wore red white and blue neckties and boys that wore fatigue hats: with girls who carry flags, and girls who carried flowers."

Fortunately, just prior to the Civil War, photography became affordable, and we are now blessed through the images assembled here to view some of the Civil War-era playtime patriots as they were attired. In post-Civil War years, children enthralled with their fathers' war stories

A TRUE CITIZEN.

continued to wear Civil War-era outfits sewn by their mothers for veterans' parades, school plays, or fun.

Playing war attired in all sorts of military uniform interpretations has never stopped. With more consumer income and cheaper manufacturing techniques available toward the end of the 19th century and the beginning of the 20th century, commercially made play military outfits and toy guns and swords became readily available. When European nations and later American soldiers were drawn into World War I, the snappy blue costumes of the Civil War and Indian Wars periods were replaced with the olive-drab wool uniforms and metal helmets of the day. Daily papers dispatching news once again called upon every nation's youth to patriotically show support by wearing all styles of uniform. When World War I ended, many uniforms were put away, but probably more were passed to the next youngest who finished them off. Prior to World War II, the period which Part One encompasses, there was no shame in playing soldier or war. My father has described chasing Indians and bad guys with his brother all over their farm during their childhood. Like men in generations before them, it was a belief in good and bad that allowed my uncle to survive a year and a half in a German POW camp and my father to survive the Korean War.

Dennis Keesee is a noted expert on Civil War boy soldiers and the author of the book *Too Young Too Die: Boy Soldiers of the Union Army 1861-1865* Blue Acorn Press, Huntington, West Virginia

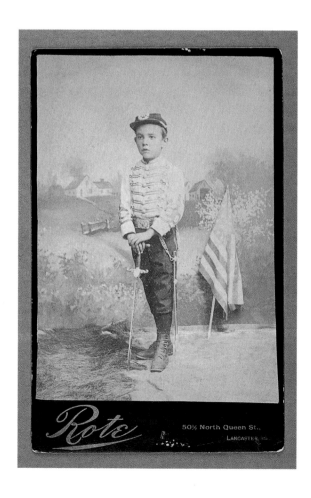

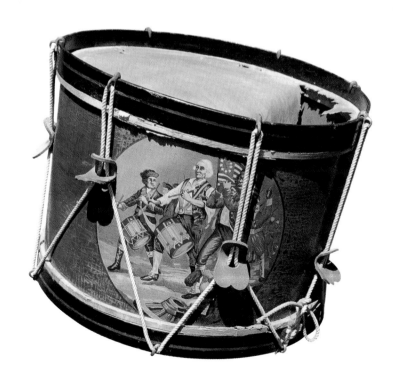

15

The Civil War Years

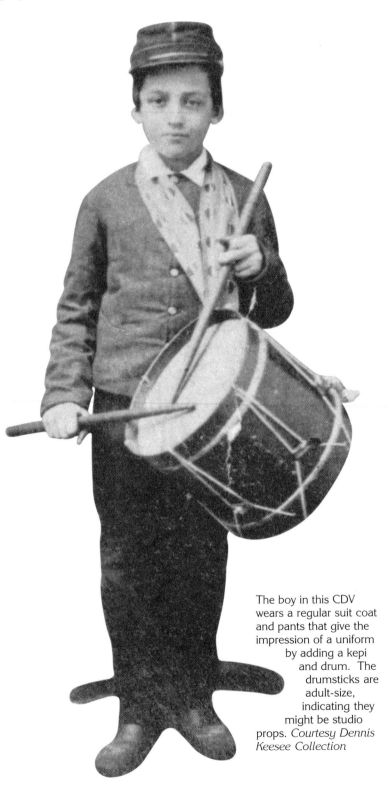

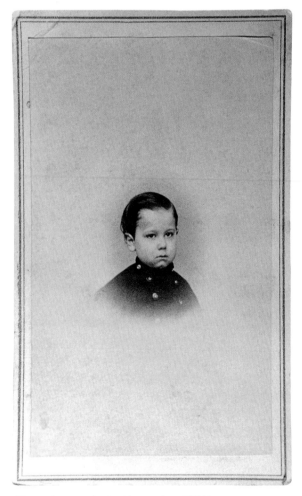

The unhappy tyke in this wartime CDV is attired in a double-breasted coat designed with what appear to be military-style buttons.

The boy in this CDV wears a regular suit coat and pants that give the impression of a uniform by adding a kepi and drum. The drumsticks are adult-size, indicating they might be studio props. *Courtesy Dennis Keesee Collection*

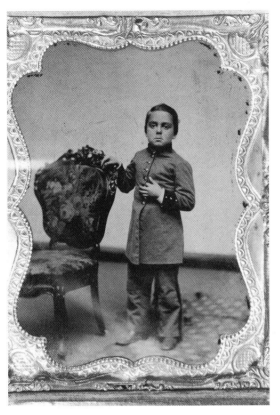

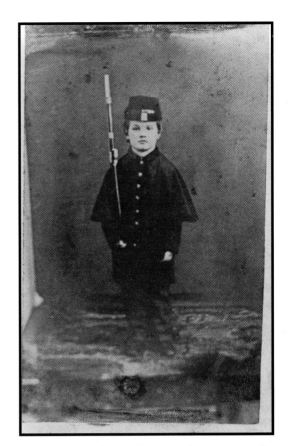

The serious young man posing in this tintype wears a coat closely tailored to a typical single-breasted frock coat worn by Federal officers and enlisted men. The pattern, first adopted in 1851, was regulation until 1872. The dark facings on the collar and cuffs might indicate branch of service, state affiliation, National Guard, or Militia. *Courtesy Dennis Keesee Collection*

It is likely this six-button "greatcoat" was patterned after an 1851 enlisted man's overcoat. His 1861-pattern forage cap and rifle fixed with a bayonet make the sell. *Courtesy Dennis Keesee Collection*

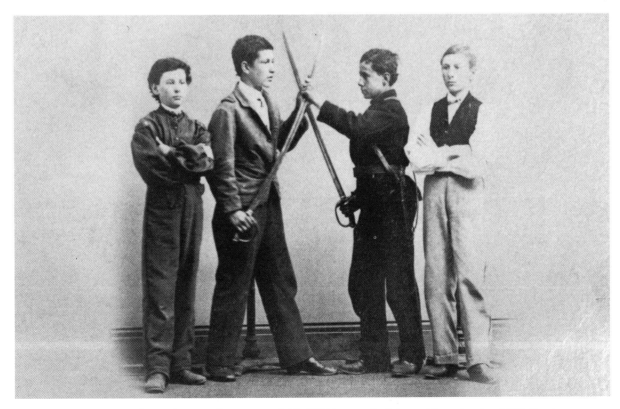

Edwin Smith, a Canton, Ohio, photographer, snapped this CDV image of adolescent boys bearing 1860 Cavalry sabers and striking a "dueling pose" with their "seconds" at their sides. *Courtesy Dennis Keesee Collection*

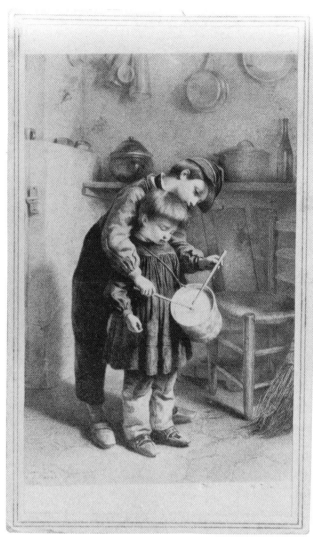

Ed Trere (artist) had his lithograph, "First Lesson on the Drum," published on CDV in 1864. *Courtesy Dennis Keesee Collection*

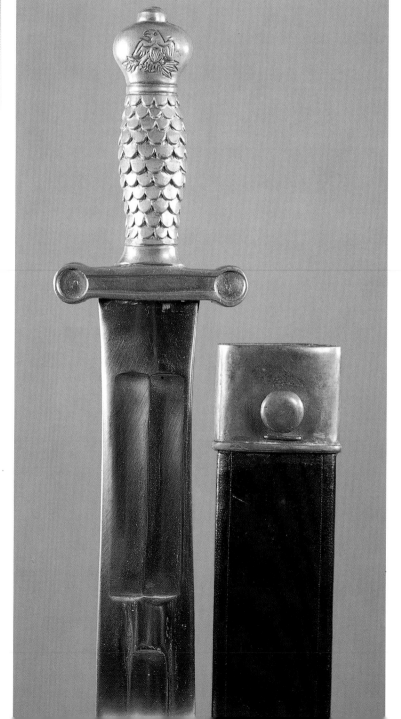

A splendid reproduction boys' version of the 1833 foot-artillery sword is exceptionally well made and true to the original. *Courtesy Man at Arms Magazine*

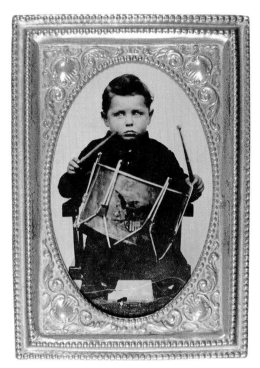

In this tintype of a very young boy photographed with an adult-size Union eagle drum, a touch of color is added to the escutcheon on the breast of the American eagle.

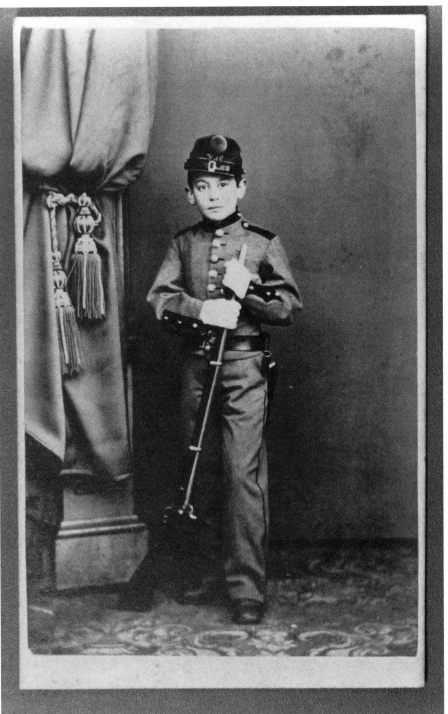

The origin of this uniform is unclear. The embroidered initials on the oval under the pompon on the hat appear to be WAC (the "C" most likely stands for Cadet[s]). The uniform is of exquisite tailoring and includes an 1839 two-piece buckle and bayonet on the belt. *Courtesy Dennis Keesee Collection*

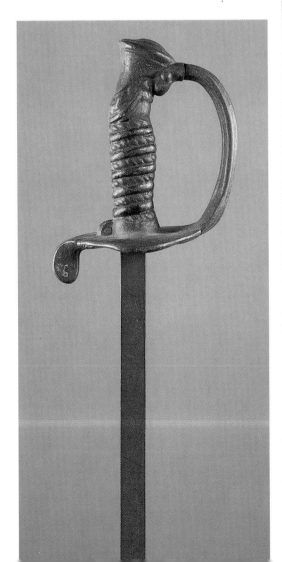

This Civil War-style boy's sword, whose style is built on either a foot-officer's or Naval-officer's pattern, has a hilt cast in two pieces and features an unusually short blade with a rounded point. *Courtesy Man at Arms Magazine*

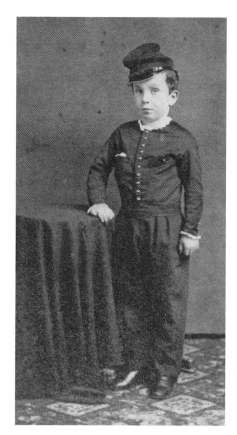

This boy wears an excellent child-size bummer-style forage cap. Headgear such as this is considered extremely rare. Few, if any, have survived. This CDV also bears the unusual McCuthan-Nevada backmark, making it collectible in more than one arena. *Courtesy Dennis Keesee Collection*

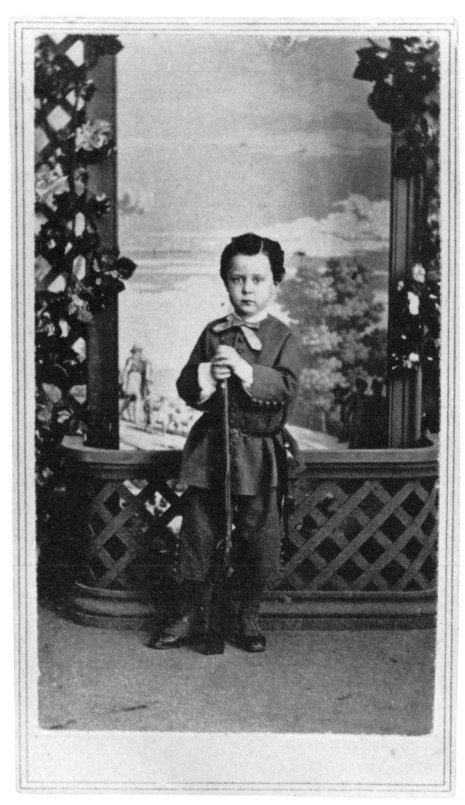

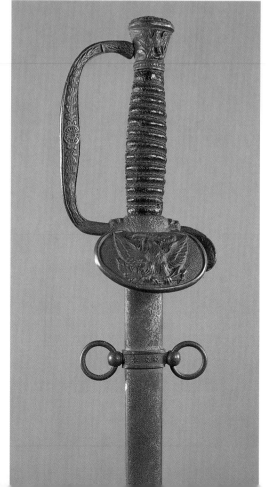

Barely visible is the boy-size Cavalry saber hanging on the hip of this junior sharpshooter. Note the fancy leggings covering his ankles and shoes. The CDV format image is backmarked C.D. Fredricks, New York, Habana, Paris. *Courtesy Dennis Keesee Collection*

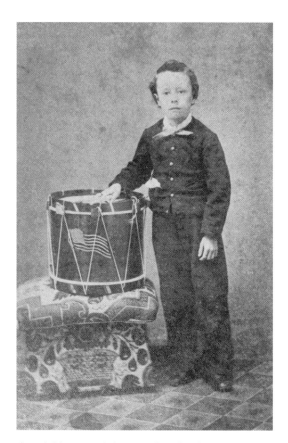

An adult's painted drum and sticks. Again, the dress suggests a military-influence cut. The addition of the kerchief around the subject's neck accentuates this further. *Courtesy Dennis Keesee Collection*

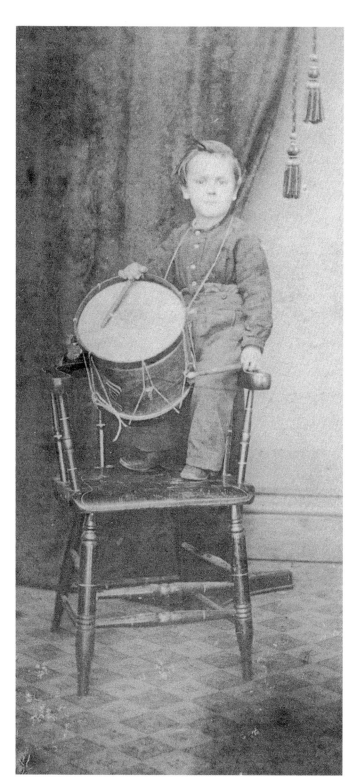

The single row of buttons on this child's belted coat faintly suggests a uniformed drummer in this CDV-format image.

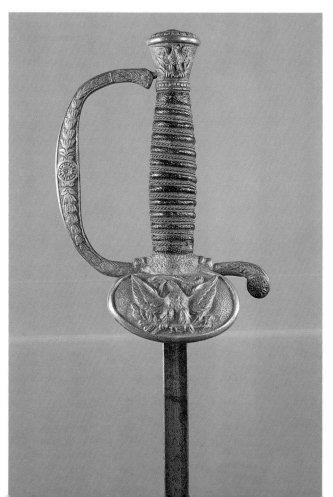

Two almost identical boys' swords are in the style of the 1860 staff and field officer's sword. *Courtesy Man at Arms Magazine*

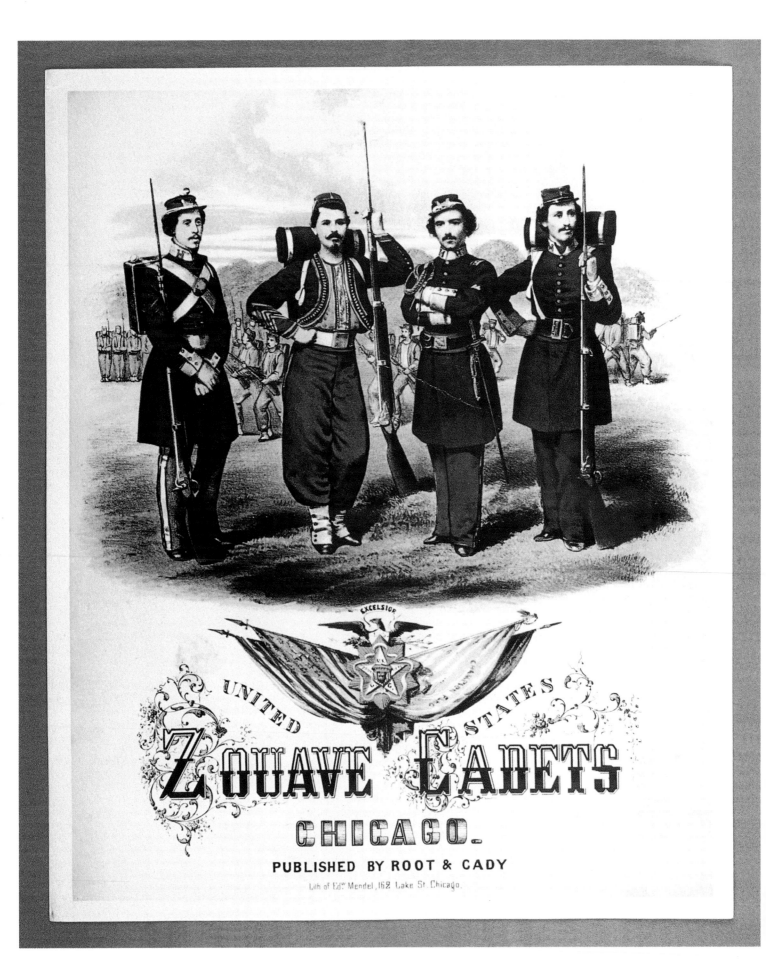

American Zouave Soldiers

The original Zouaves were North Africans (mainly Kabyles [Berbers]) of the Zouaua tribe who offered their military services to occupying French troops when they captured the city of Algiers in early 1830.

Over the next few years some occupying French abandoned their traditional military dress, accepting the more Arabic-influenced dress of the North Africans, which consisted of loose, baggy trousers; open jackets; and fezzes for headgear. More suitably dressed for the desert climate, they became the first of the French Zouave regiments.

The American Zouaves (The United States Zouave Cadets) were founded by Colonel Elmer E. Ellsworth of Chicago, Illinois, who envisioned an American take on the Imperial French Guard. The all-volunteer group soon gained fame for its exotic dress, elaborate military drill, and gymnastic antics. Local popularity quickly became national notoriety when Ellsworth took the troop on a tour of the Eastern U.S. to challenge other volunteer militia groups to displays of military mastery and competence. The idea was a success, and soon everyone was talking about the Zouaves.

With the threat of secession by southern states and Civil War imminent, volunteer groups from both northern and southern states formed regiments of Zouaves and readied for battle. Individual groups designed their own interpretation of Zouave dress.

Some groups adopted the traditional Imperial French Guard uniform with little deviation. Others chose to incorporate elements of the traditional dress into their existing uniforms. Eventually, most units had a common thread identifying them as Zouave units—woolen open-front jacket and distinctive cloverleaf design sewn to the breast and sleeves, known as *tombeau*.

For children, in contrast, the suddenly fashionable Zouave style was less structured and defined than its adult counterpart. A sort of pseudo-Zouave fashion appeared that implemented a broader interpretation, utilizing multicolors and fabric choices. But like the adult version, the identifying trait was almost always the open-front jacket.

As the Civil War raged, children in northern states were soon hauled to photographers for portraits featuring the broadly interpreted and trendy Zouave fashions. So common, in fact, was the uniformed boy during the 1860s, that an English visitor to New York commented acidly that, from the deck of his arriving ship, the docks of the city seemed to be populated by "organ grinders' monkeys."

Zouave fashion for children continued in popularity through the end of the war, receding into obscurity as quickly as it appeared less than five years earlier.

This song sheet illustrates three of the original uniforms of the United States Zouave Cadets, 1860. *Courtesy Michael J. McAfee*

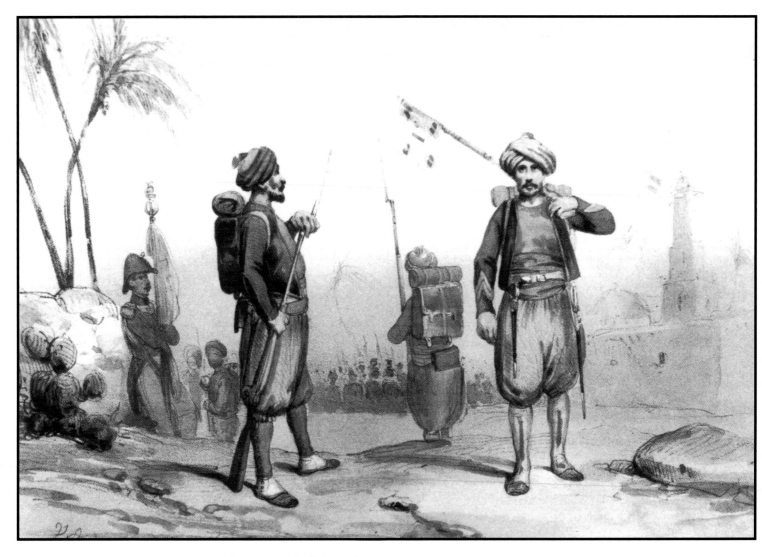

The French Zouaves in Algiers, 1832. *Courtesy Michael J. McAfee*

In this image taken on April 1, 1865, a young Zouave draws his Cavalry saber from its scabbard, readying for combat. *Courtesy Dennis Keesee Collection*

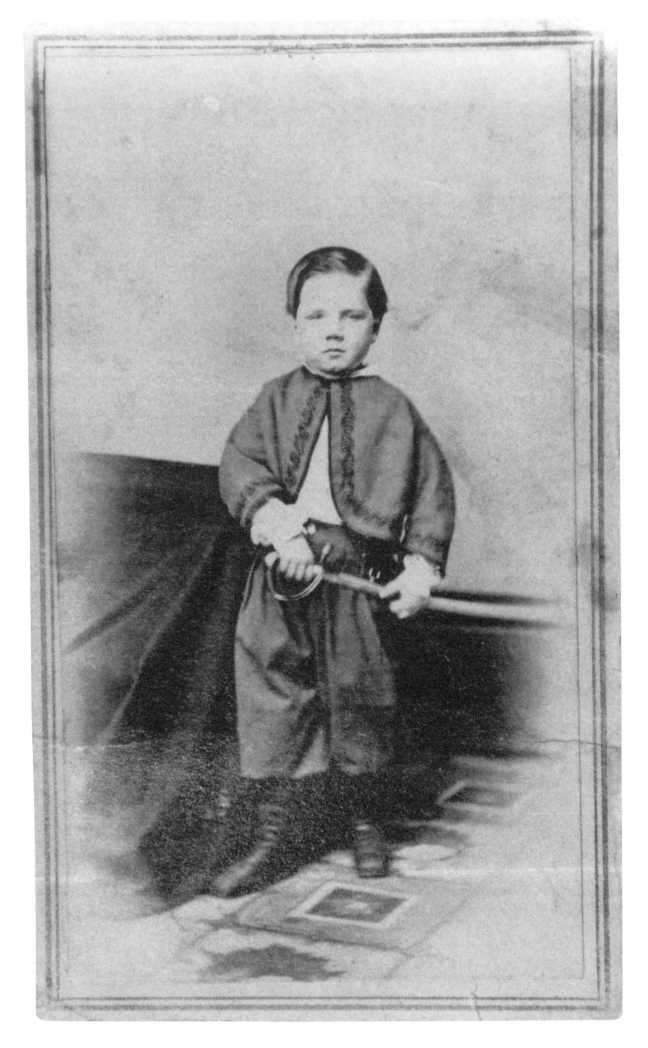

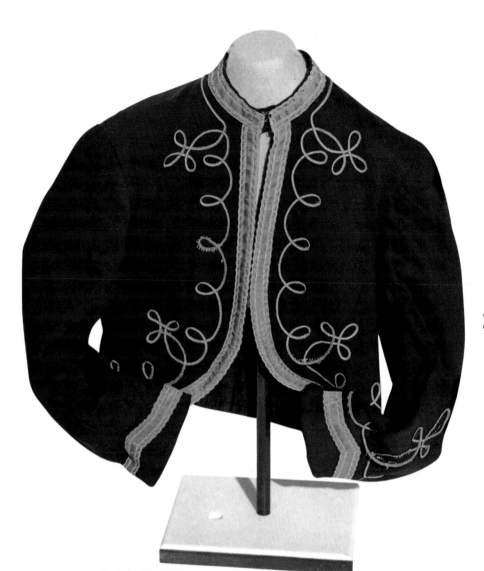

A post-war Zouave jacket for a boy of about eleven or twelve years old.

Many elements in this CDV make it desirable. The most obvious is the hint of military style, but the not-quite-so-obvious elements are that the child is in a reclining position and he is barefoot. Both these factors are quite unusual for this period. *Courtesy Jerry Mulholland*

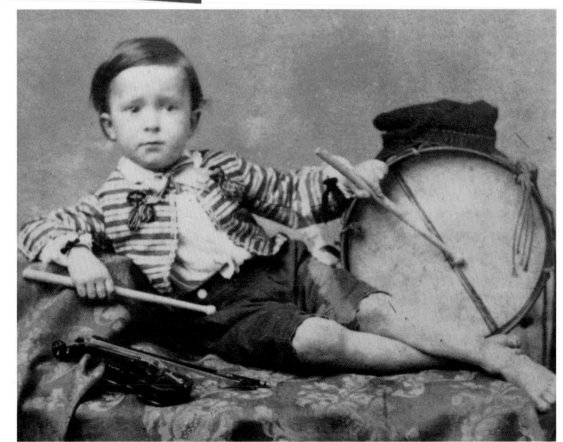

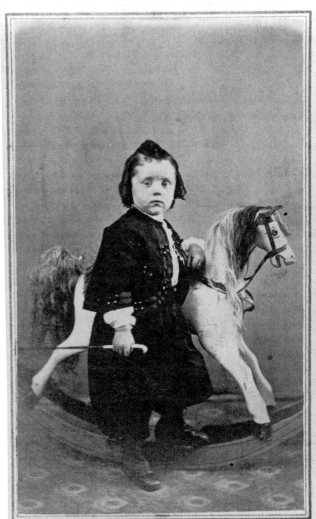

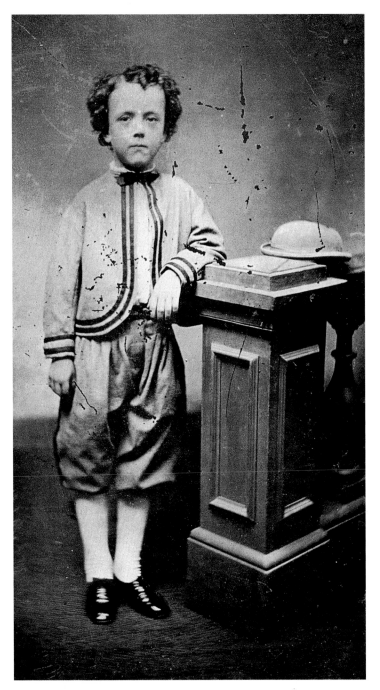

The Zouave skin-horse soldier in this CDV wields a boy-size riding crop. *Courtesy Dennis Keesee Collection*

The telltale white stockings, baggy trousers, and open-front decorated jacket of the Zouaves have evolved into fashion of the day. A non-military-style hat perches on the pedestal.

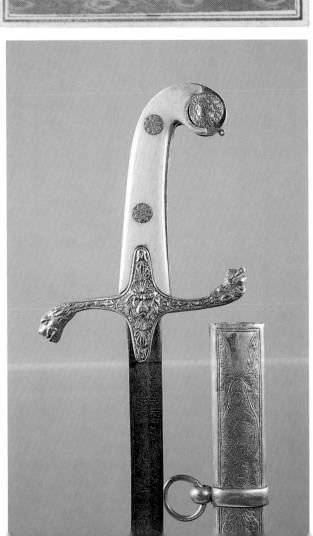

The English-style Mameluke officer's sword has been shortened for use by a boy. The deeply etched blade features a variety of military devices. The scabbard, in addition to being shortened, has had the drag remounted to complete the effect (not shown). The ricasso is marked with a K&C and a king's head next to an armored head, indicating manufacture in Solingen by Weyersberg, Kirschbaum & Company. *Courtesy Man at Arms Magazine*

Boys of this era relished the idea of being captured in images as brave soldiers, and dreamed of marching off with a regiment to bear the colors or beat the drum.

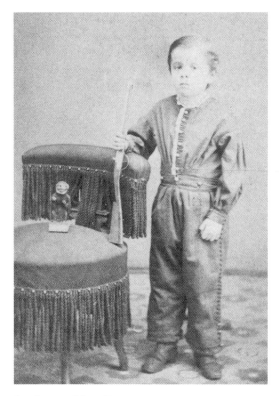

A solemn soldier. *Courtesy Dennis Keesee Collection*

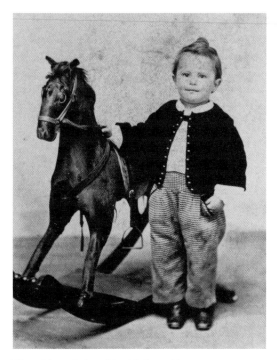

The wide waistband in this broad interpretation suggests a trait of many Zouave-styled trousers—the trademark sash. *Courtesy Dennis Keesee Collection*

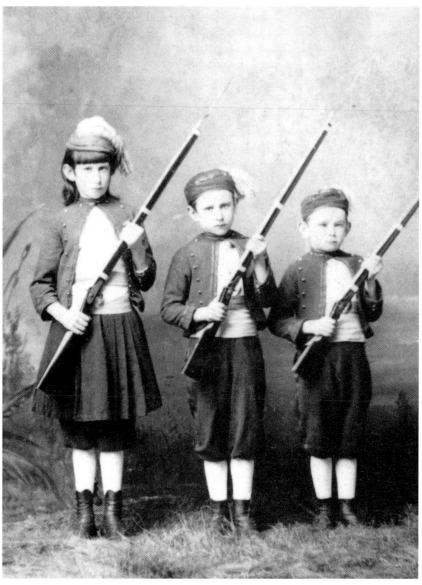

An extraordinary studio CDV of three siblings in full Zouave regalia. With such attention to detail, it is likely they have strong ties to a soldier serving in a Zouave regiment. Their true Imperial Guard-style uniforms are complete with white leggings and sashes that cover the tops of their trousers. The two boys appear to have turban-wrapped fezzes (chechia), and the to-scale period weapons make this image exceptional. *Courtesy Steve Lister*

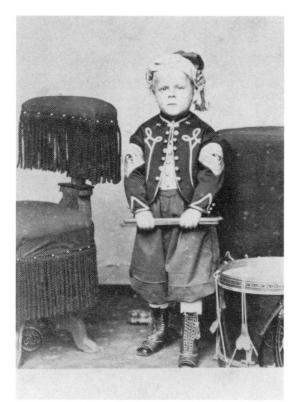

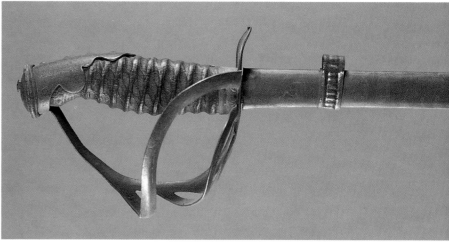

Civil War officer-style sword of spectacularly low quality. *Courtesy Man at Arms Magazine*

This mass-produced CDV carries the unusual Barnum & Bailey (circus) tax stamp dated 4-26-(18)66. The studio backmark is E. and H.T. Anthony, whose photographic studio was renowned for its images of well-known personalities. The boy shown in this image was a drumming prodigy recruited by Barnum as part of a troop he formed called Infant Drummers of the Civil War. Note the exaggerated shoulder insignia and the hem on his Zouave trousers, which have been let down, most likely to accommodate a growth spurt. For a child billed as an "infant," and growing quickly, time was a factor working against the novelty of this boy's career and Barnum's pocketbook. *Courtesy Dennis Keesee Collection*

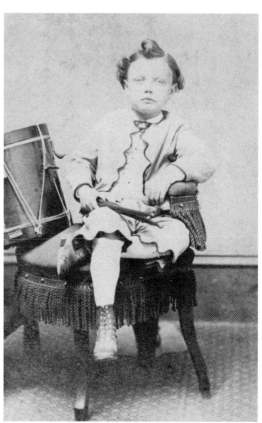

The scalloped edges on the jacket and trouser hem are a good example of the liberties taken in boys' Zouave fashion. *Courtesy Dennis Keesee Collection*

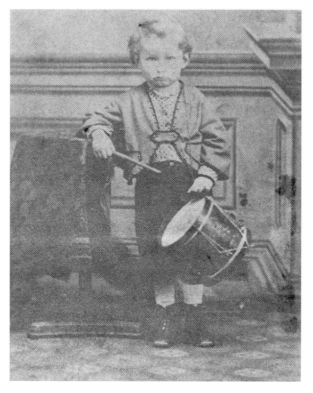

The ball buttons decorating the edge of the open-front jacket are, by design, similar to the style used by the 95th Pennsylvania, Goslin's Zouaves. *Courtesy Dennis Keesee Collection*

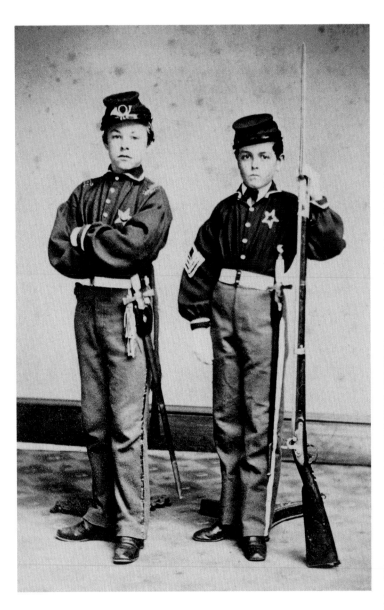

A remarkably accurate image with plenty of attention to detail. Wearing bummer-style kepis, the subject on the left bears an 1858 infantry horn. Militia-style (1850s) swords and stars on their blouses indicate 12th or 20th affiliation (Army Corps Badges). Note that the uniforms are obviously adult-size. The boy on the right wears a chevron shoulder patch that nearly reaches to his elbow. Copious amounts of blouse tucked into the front of the trousers give both quite a bulge below the belt. The swords are 1840 to 1850s Militia. *Courtesy Dennis Keesee Collection*

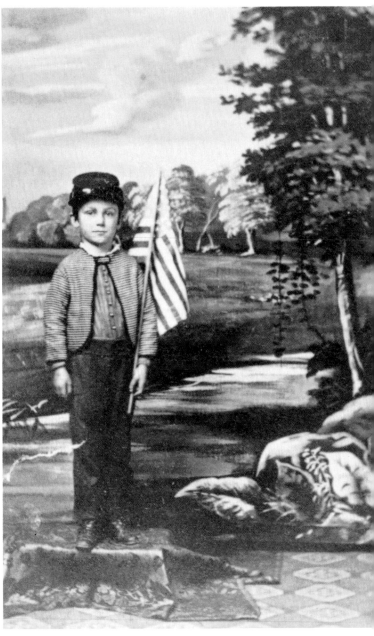

Flags were a favorite prop, making a seemingly common studio background suddenly patriotic. *Courtesy Fred Jolly*

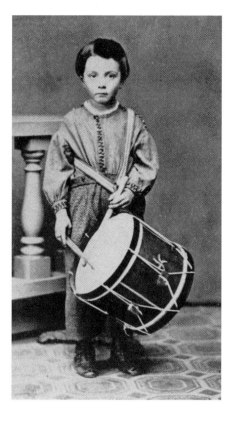

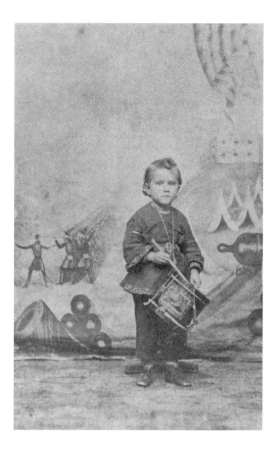

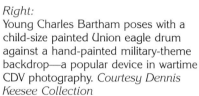

Left:
Without the drum, the liberal Zouave influence of this boy's outfit might be mistaken for a common playsuit. *Courtesy Dennis Keesee Collection*

Right:
Young Charles Bartham poses with a child-size painted Union eagle drum against a hand-painted military-theme backdrop—a popular device in wartime CDV photography. *Courtesy Dennis Keesee Collection*

In this CDV, two boys sport adult-size uniforms exaggerating the Zouave style with oversized rank. These outfits were likely part of a studio's costume collection. The heavy loads they carry are a bass drum and an 1840 officer's sword. The overall package makes this image highly desirable and collectible. *Courtesy Dennis Keesee Collection*

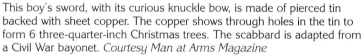

This boy's sword, with its curious knuckle bow, is made of pierced tin backed with sheet copper. The copper shows through holes in the tin to form 6 three-quarter-inch Christmas trees. The scabbard is adapted from a Civil War bayonet. *Courtesy Man at Arms Magazine*

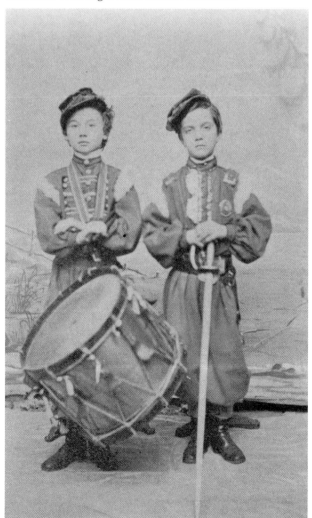

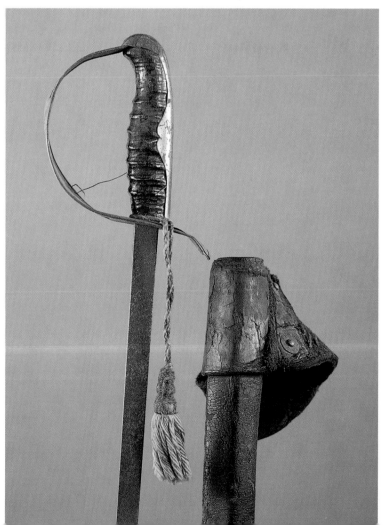

Celebrating America's Centennial—

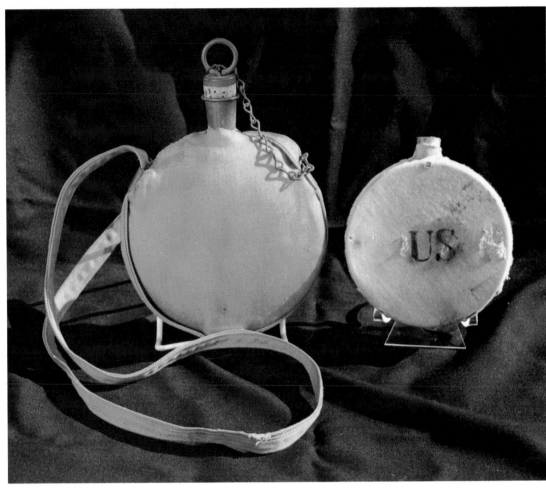

Two post-Civil War children's canteens. The style on the left remained largely unchanged until around the turn of the century when strap adjusters were added.

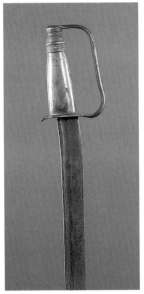

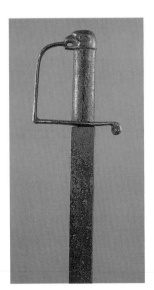

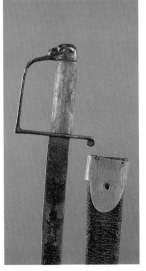

A primitive American boy's sword (left) features an interesting crudely fullered blade and cast-brass grip that appears to have been made from an as-yet-unidentified object. Early-19th-century American eagle hilted boys' swords (center and right) were obviously produced in significant numbers. These were made in the United States, which is quite a rarity. The sword in this view is distinct in that it is fitted with a scabbard cut down from an adult version.
Courtesy Man at Arms Magazine

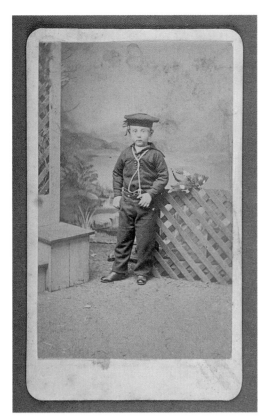

This lad looks surly and dressed beyond his years as a sailor. Young boys of the era were employed on Naval vessels as "powder monkeys" (boys who brought munitions to gun loaders on ships). The CDV, dated Oct 2, 1870, is backmarked W.M. Shew, a famous San Francisco photographer.

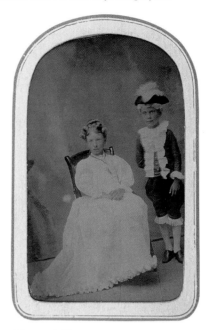

These children wear costumes honoring heroes of the American Revolution such as George and Martha Washington, as in the photo lower right in this Centennial-period tintype.

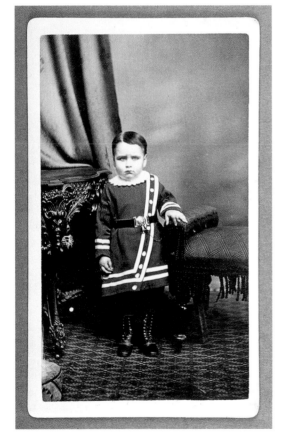

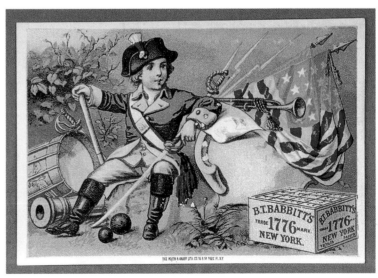

A child in a patriotic dress and two-piece, lion-head belt plate. Members of the British Army, circa 1860 to 1870s, wore this type of belt plate. It has been suggested through battlefield recoveries that some of these may have been imported by blockade runners and saw limited use by Confederate troops.

This lithograph of a young boy depicts a fully equipped Revolutionary in a B.T. Babbitt's Soap advertisement. The back of the card reads: "Worth ten times its cost to every mother and family in Christendom."

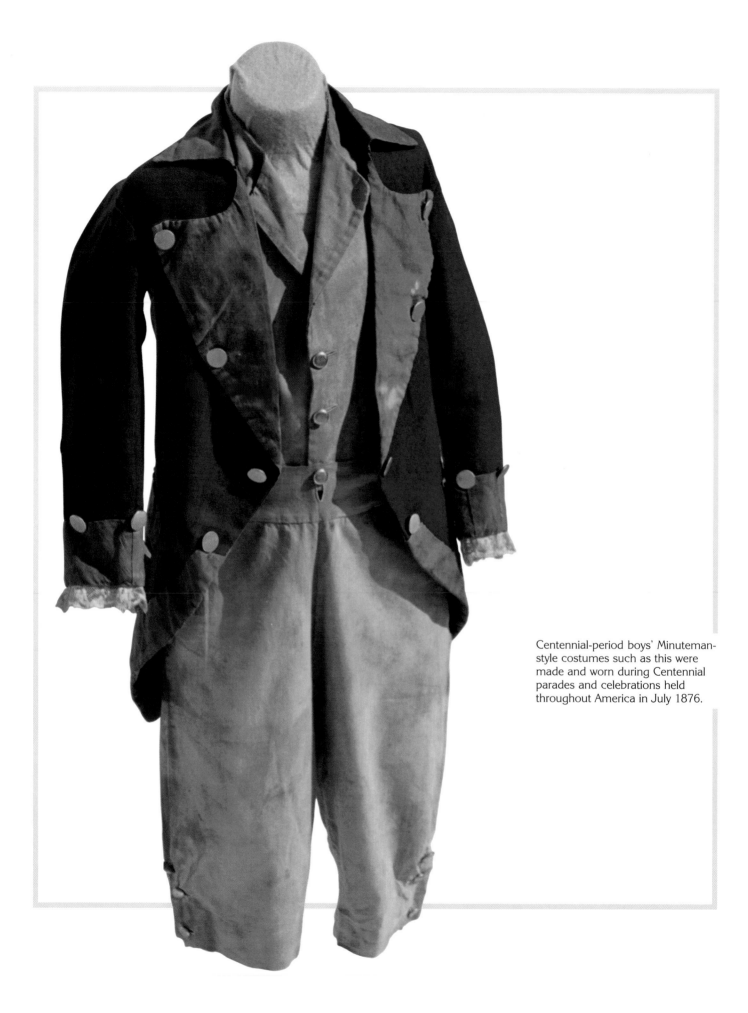

Centennial-period boys' Minuteman-style costumes such as this were made and worn during Centennial parades and celebrations held throughout America in July 1876.

Since photography did not exist during the American Revolutionary era, people relied on drawings, paintings, and verbal accounts of period dress. This Minuteman has several accurate characteristics of period costume, including his 1751 British-pattern-style infantry sword. Note the powdered wig under the tricorn hat.

An American boy's saber features a unique but crude pattern. One-of-a-kind examples such as this would have been commonplace during the period but are hard to find today. They vary widely in quality of construction, ranging from delicate toys to dangerous weapons. Some may have been fabricated from existing blades by family members, but it is unlikely that many survived the rough play of childhood war games. Most would have been discarded or passed on to another child. *Courtesy Man at Arms Magazine*

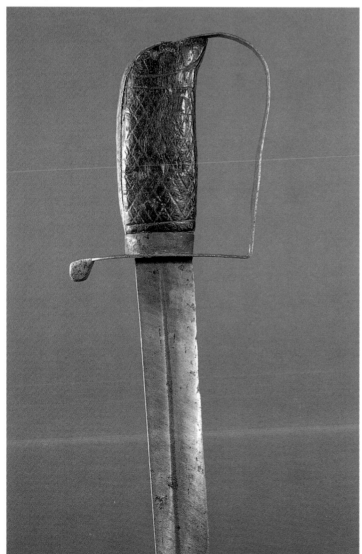

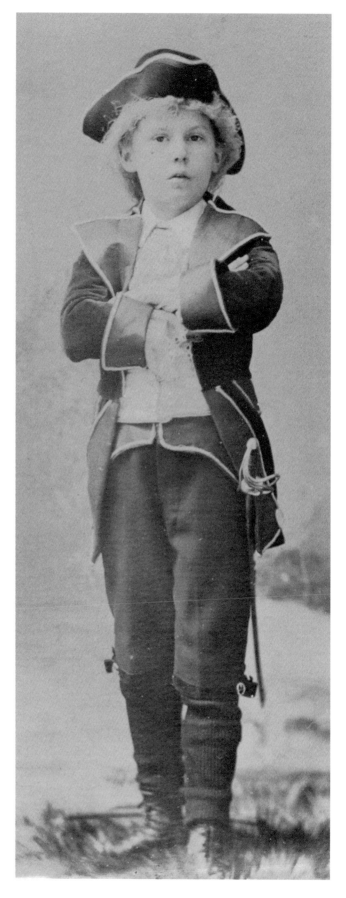

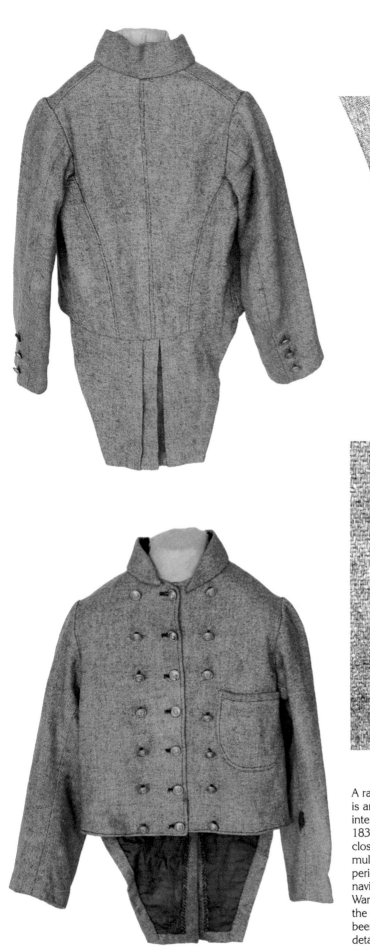

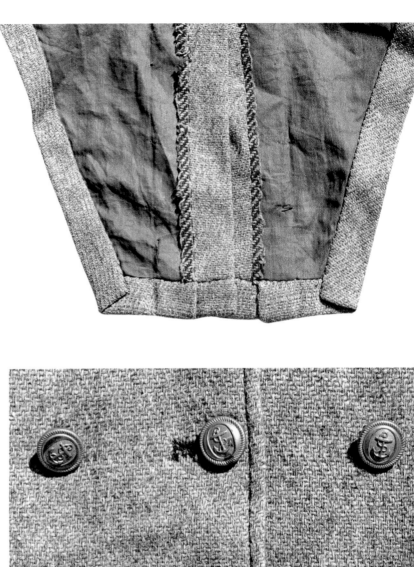

A rare triple breasted child's coat that was discovered in Norfolk, Virginia, is an excellent example of how adult military uniform characteristics were interpreted for children's fashion. Though it is likely that this Coatee (style 1830-1880) was manufactured during the later half of the 1870s, it closely parallels the earlier patterns of pre-Civil War Southern Militias. Its multipiece cut and the polished cotton lining are consistent with the period and the tin-back buttons are representative of the style used by navies of the world at the time. The outer fabric is considered to be Civil War-era loom-woven lindsey-woolsey, and with the exposed binding on the inside of the coattails, it would be easy to believe this coat might have been cut from a Confederate blanket. Because of the close attention to detail, one may conclude that the sewer had considerable uniform tailoring experience.

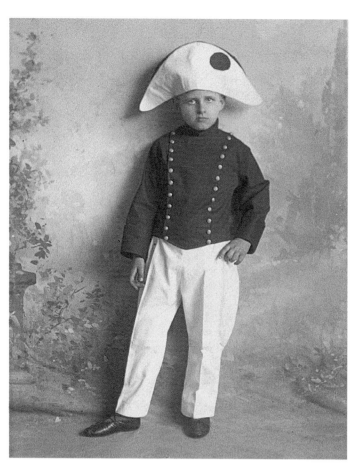

In this photograph of an 1870s French CDV, the boy wears a Napoleonic-period-style uniform.

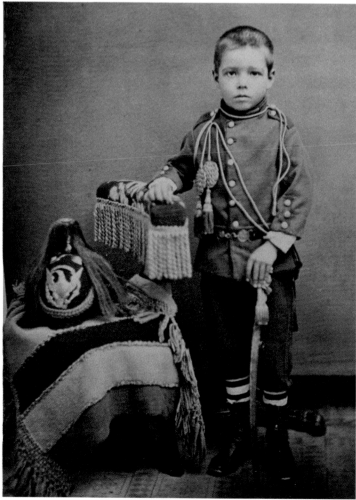

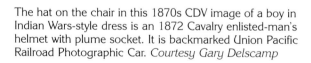

The hat on the chair in this 1870s CDV image of a boy in Indian Wars-style dress is an 1872 Cavalry enlisted-man's helmet with plume socket. It is backmarked Union Pacific Railroad Photographic Car. *Courtesy Gary Delscamp*

After the Battles

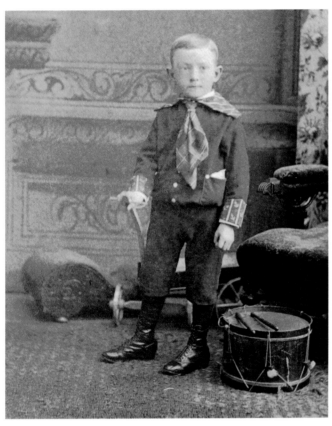

The bib collar, tie, and cuffs in an anchor pattern may have been made separately and added to the suit just for the photograph. *Courtesy Terri Stewart Collection*

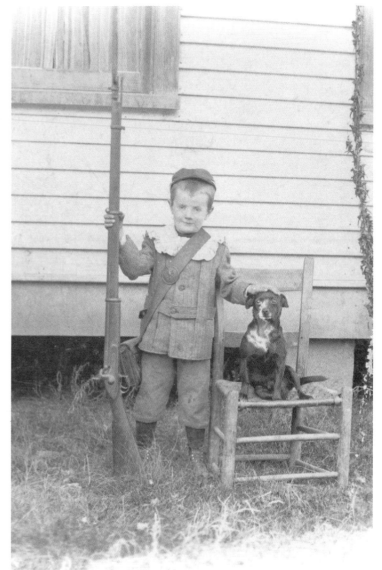

This circa 1880s cabinet card shows a small boy holding a British-made 1853 Enfield rifled musket and a .58 caliber cartridge box bearing the familiar eagle plate. The cartridge box was standard issue to Union troops during the Civil War. This type rifle was issued to several Union regiments, most notably the 44th Massachusetts. *Courtesy Dennis Keesee Collection*

Finely detailed child's stamped-brass officers' waist belt plate in the 1851 pattern. Notably, the popularity of this design was prescribed in U.S. Army regulations through 1941, with only minor changes to the pattern and belt attachment.

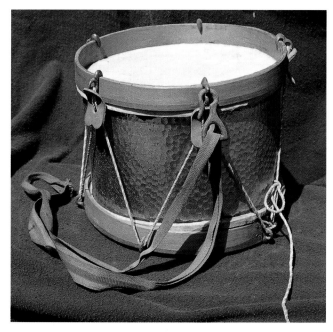

Circa 1890s Noble & Cooley hammered-brass child's drum with sling. *Courtesy Noble & Cooley Co.*

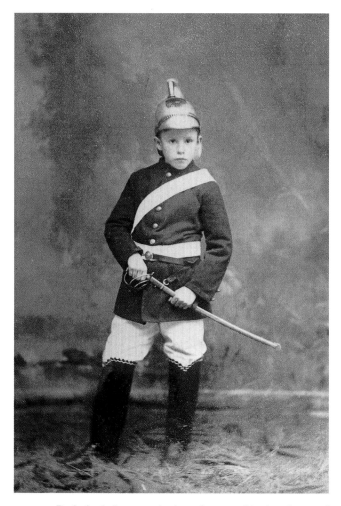

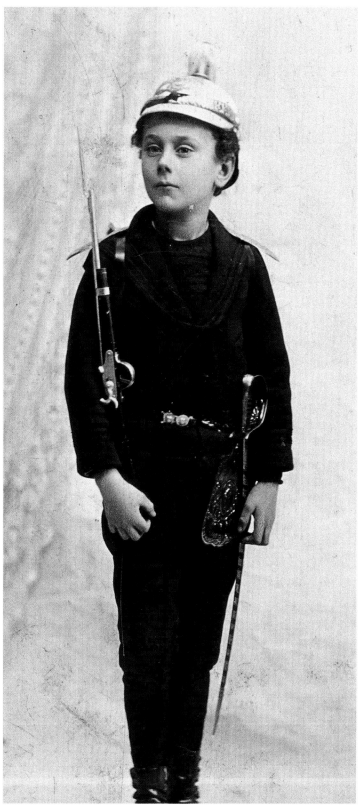

Both the helmet on the boy above and in the photo right vaguely represent the style of an American 1881 helmet with plume socket, with regulation-specified use by mounted troops. Spikes on American helmets were worn by foot soldiers. *Photo above Courtesy Michael J. Bremer Collection*

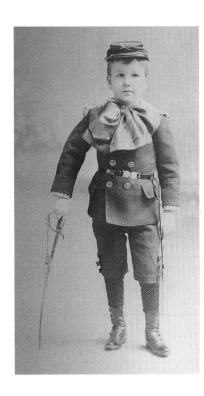

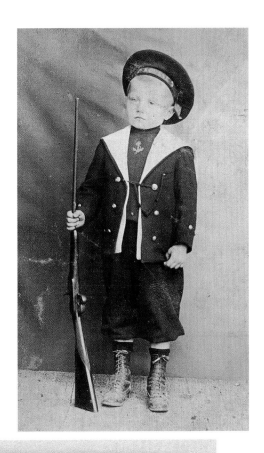

Left:
This handsome soldier has a wonderful two-piece buckle (unidentified) on his sword belt, which holds the scabbard of his drawn sword. A bow was a popular accessory in boys' fashion during the American late-Victorian period. The cabinet card photography is by Ferson & Williams, Columbus, Ohio.

Right:
Maroon-faced cabinet cards such as these date in the 1880s. The tally on this French sailor's cap reads "Toulouse." In the 19th century, each French unit was attached to a particular city or port in the French republic (for example, Bretagne, Navarre, and Bourgogre are towns and cities in France that have had Naval units bear their names).

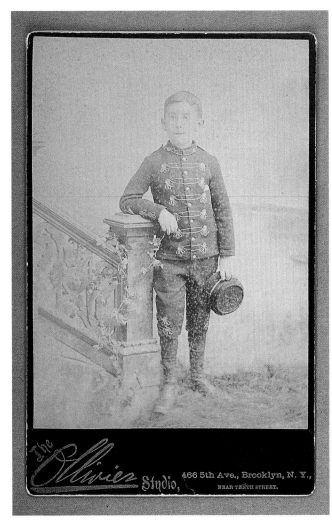

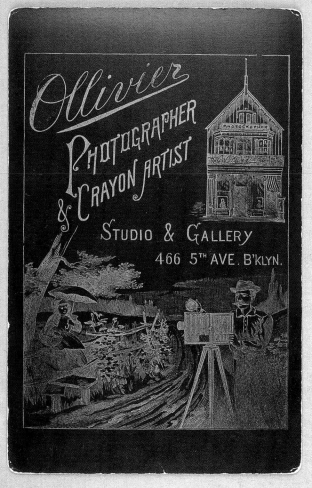

The extra-fancy interpretation of this military-style uniform makes quite an impression; however, the photographer's beautiful backmark on this 1880s cabinet card rivals the subject on the front.

"Fellow-Citizens: We stand today upon an eminence which overlooks a hundred years of national life – a century with perils, but crowned with the triumphs of liberty and law. Before continuing the onward march let us pause on this height for a moment to strengthen our faith and renew our hope by a glance at a pathway along which our people have traveled."

Inaugural address of President James Garfield, March 4, 1881. He was mortally wounded by an assassin four months later.

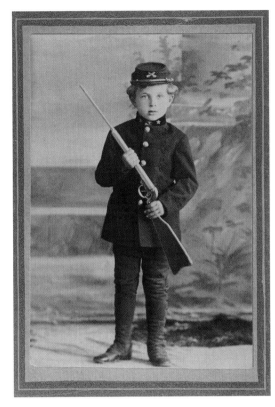

This boy wears the same coat as the one shown right. Although the coat is an 1888 pattern, the 3rd model Daisy wasn't introduced until 1895, dating this image later than a first glance might indicate.

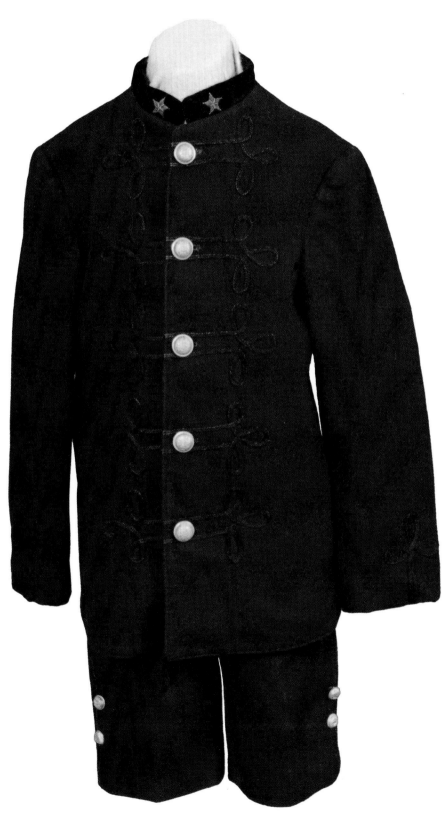

A beautifully preserved 1888-pattern Army uniform tailored in New York. The coat and knee-length trousers are made of high-quality wool. Black collar and black mohair quatrefoil, as well as the bullion stars and button style, would make it general's staff.

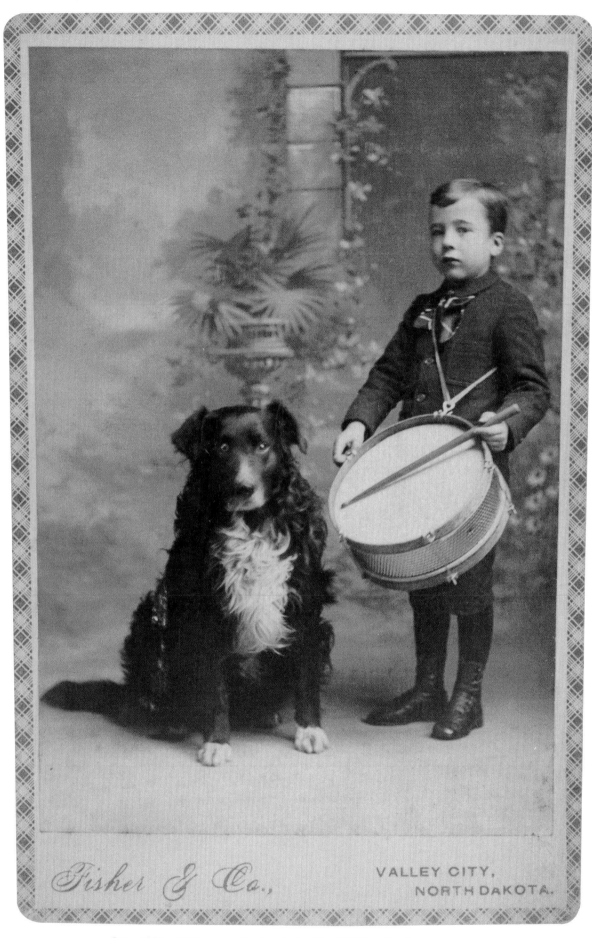

Fisher & Co., VALLEY CITY,
NORTH DAKOTA.

Circa 1890s. Thirty years after the start of the Civil War, the drum maintains its prominence in children's photography. *Courtesy Adele Gilmore*

Noble & Cooley Co.

In January 1854, Silas Noble and James P. Cooley started making drums in the Noble's farmhouse kitchen. Their drum was an immediate success. In a few weeks they moved into a small building and after two years built their first factory. In 1860, from a rail split by Abraham Lincoln, Noble & Cooley Co. made a drum used in political rallies in Massachusetts and Connecticut. This drum was presented to the 10th Massachusetts Regiment and eventually found a resting place in the United States Patent Office.

During the Civil War the company boomed, so to speak, making drums for Union regiments, expanding to a larger factory, and eventually switching from the use of waterpower to steam engine. A few years later the company produced the largest drum on record, an eight-foot-diameter behemoth made especially for use in Boston in 1868 during the Ulysses S. Grant presidential campaign. Later it was used in the 1876 Centennial.

Noble & Cooley Co. not only made military drums of all sizes but also toy drums. In 1854 the company produced 631 drums. By 1873 it was manufacturing 100,000 drums per year.

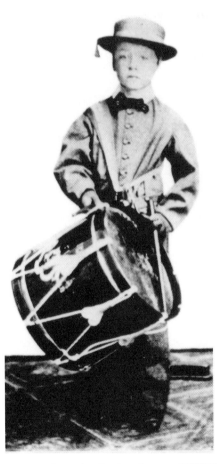

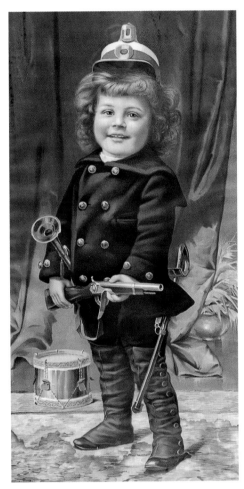

"The Home Guard" is a lovely Victorian print that hangs in the offices at Noble & Cooley. A closer look (below) reveals tiny print inside the rim of the drum that reads: "Copyright 1891- The Great Atlantic Pacific Tea Company, New York." The drum in the print is a representation of a Noble & Cooley toy drum of the era. *Courtesy Noble & Cooley Co.*

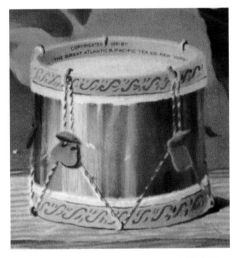

A cousin from the Cooley clan poses with a drum from the family business. *Courtesy Noble & Cooley Co.*

A trio of patriotic-design toy drums from the collection of vintage drums displayed in the executive office at Noble & Cooley Co. go back over 100 years. *Courtesy Noble & Cooley Co.*

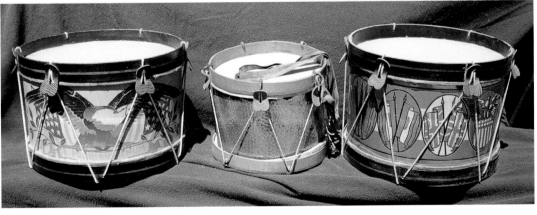

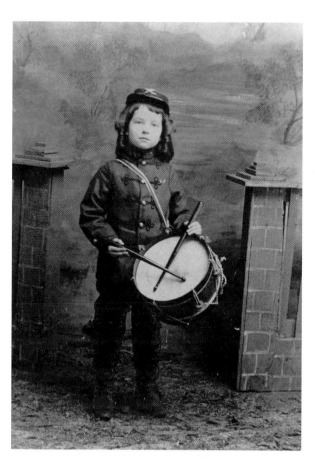

The back of this photo reads: "Laura McKinny, near nine years old, in the same room with Kaley at school, played drummer boy in 'Battle of Shiloh' at Opera House Fri & Sat nights Feb 17-18-99. (1899)." The "Drummer Boy of Shilioh, or The Battlefield of Shiloh, a new Military Allegory in Five Acts and a Comp Tableaux," was published in 1872 by Conrad Samuel J. Muscroft. The post-Civil War national tour of "Shiloh" paved the way for many local chapters of the G.A.R., which produced the play locally to raise funds during the 1880s and 1890s for G.A.R. events and soldiers' homes. Note the low profile of the subject's kepi. This is actually an 1872-pattern forage cap and not the 1858 pattern, which was used during the Civil War. *Courtesy Dennis Keesee Collection*

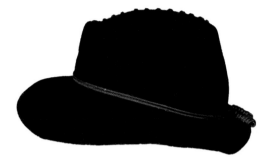

A child's version of a non-regulation campaign or "slouch" hat personifies the image of the Rebel soldier. This late-19th-century example has a laced peak. Campaign hats enjoyed long service with the U.S. Army until 1940. State Militias were eventually absorbed by State Guard Units.

The sword at left, circa 1892, is marked on the ricasso "E.A. Armstrong/Manufacturing Company/141-3 Wabash Ave./Chicago." The obverse of the ricasso bears a stamp in the shape of an unidentified rodent or forest animal. The blade is light etched with foliation, and a U.S. and American eagle holding a ribbon reads "E. Pluribus Unum." The Armstrong Company of Chicago was one of the premier suppliers of military goods in 19th-century America. The boy's sword in the image at right is a French pattern. The blade etching features an American eagle with a ribbon reading "E. Pluribus Unum" on the reverse and the boy's name on the obverse. *Courtesy Man at Arms Magazine*

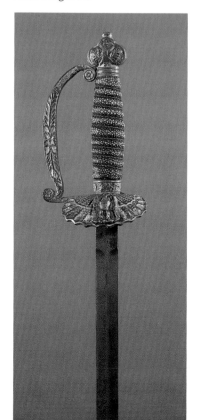

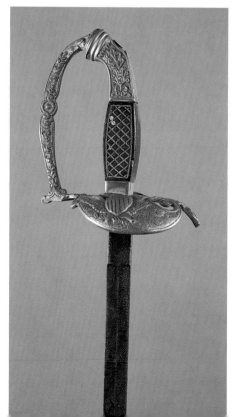

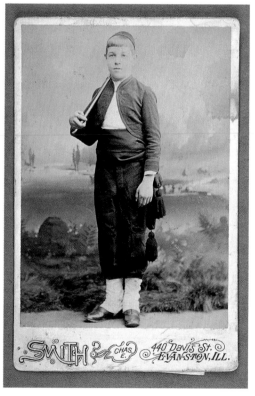

Federal Zouave units were disbanded after the Civil War; however, Zouave Militia units existed in America up to World War I. In this cabinet card image dated 1888, the young man is dressed in a homemade uniform and may have had ties to a family member in a state Militia unit. State Militia Units were eventually absorbed into State Guard Units.

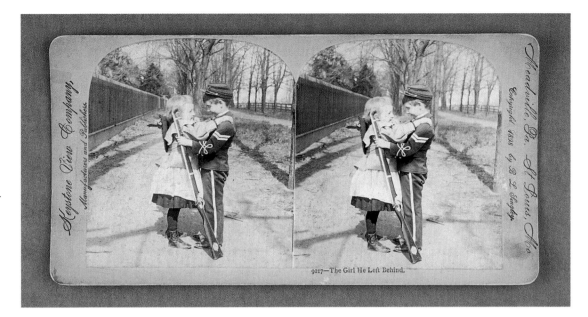

Keystone View Company published a series of stereo-view cards of children in military dress in a variety of adult poses. The one at right, "The Girl He Left Behind," is copyrighted 1898 by B.L. Singley.

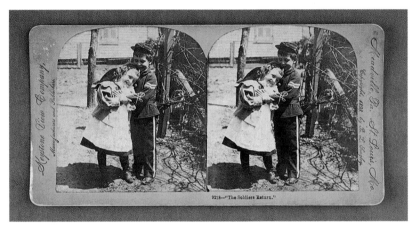

The next view in the series is called "The Soldiers Return."

This view was copyrighted in 1902 by T.W. Ingersoll and is captioned "None but the Brave Deserve the Fair." The back of the card gives a romantic description of a soldier's return from war: "When Charles V. entered Antwerp, the belles of that ancient city are said to have gone forth nude to greet him: when Hobson had corked up the harbor of Santiago, he was rewarded by showers of kisses by American women. Hero worship has been innate in women ever from times ages ago, when man's existence was a series of fights with wild beasts and savage foes, when his defeat meant perdition or slavery for his dear ones, and when every safe return home was an occasion for thanksgiving and love's reward. It is her feminine instinct that drives Nellie into the arms of the bold warrior to rest her head blissfully on his manly bosom."

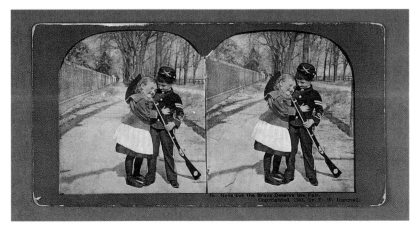

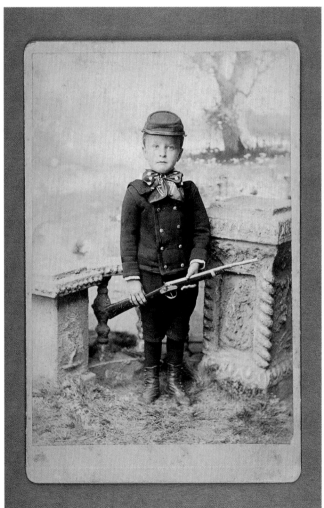

An unidentified cabinet card-format image of a boy in an 1872-style forage cap. The bullion chinstrap across the brim would indicate officer status.

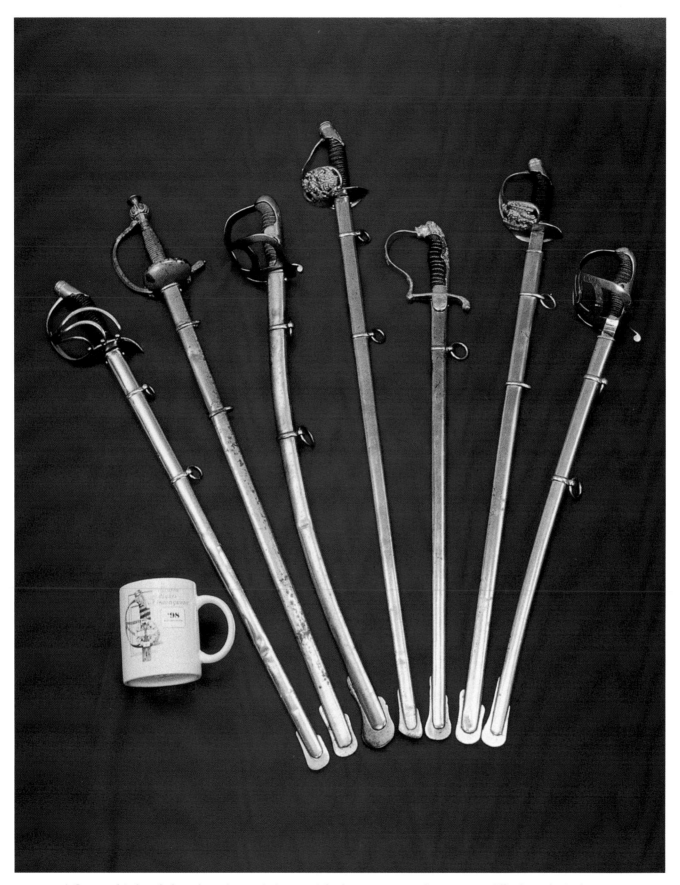

A German *kindersabel* can be quite rare in its own right, but some examples are more difficult to obtain than others. In general, those saber patterns that are rare in their large counterpart are ultra-rare in *kindersabel* size. Shown left to right are heavy mounted Cavalry design with nickel scabbard, civil or court *degan* with nickel scabbard, highly curved 1851 Cavalry saber with nickel scabbard, Model 1889 Würtemberg Infantry *degan* with nickel scabbard, lion-head *degan* with generic crossguard and straight scabbard, Model 1889 Prussian Infantry *degan* with nickel scabbard, and 1851 Cavalry saber with nickel scabbard. *Courtesy Marie DiMartini Whittmann Collection. Photo: Charles Jenkins, III*

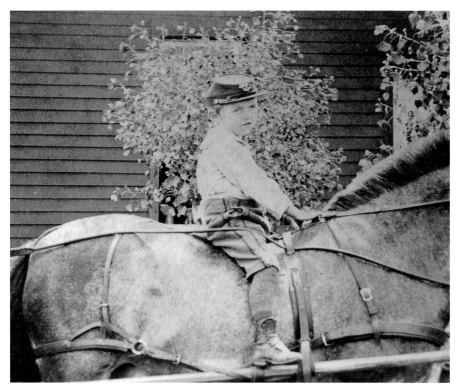

A young mounted soldier. *Courtesy Terri Stewart Collection*

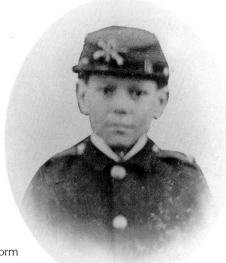

A silhouette portrait of a boy in a uniform and kepi with 1876-style insignia.

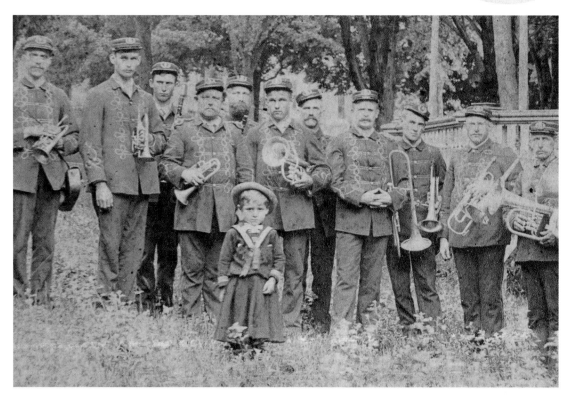

The kepis worn by the musicians in this pre-Spanish-American War photo are in the 1895 pattern. The little mascot is wearing a wonderful patriotic dress and cap in this large-format cabinet card image.

To Hell with Spain, Remember the Maine!

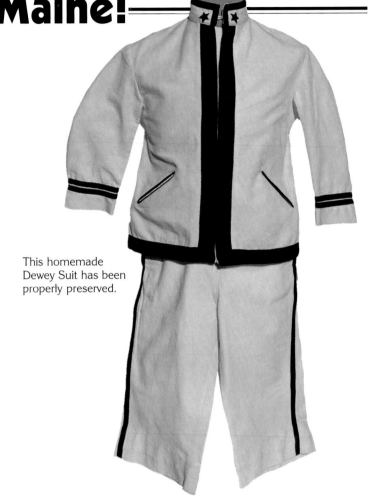

This homemade Dewey Suit has been properly preserved.

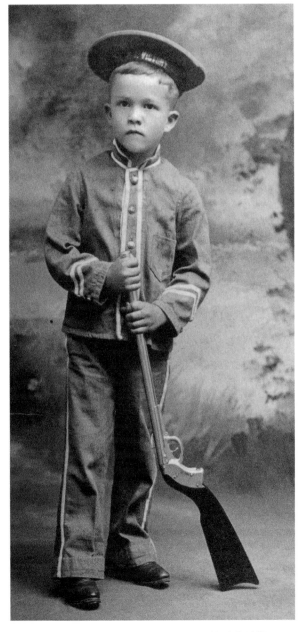

A boy in a Dewey Suit holds a New King Model 1895 B.B. gun. The photographer is Jackson, Middlebury, Vermont. *Courtesy Michael J. Bremer*

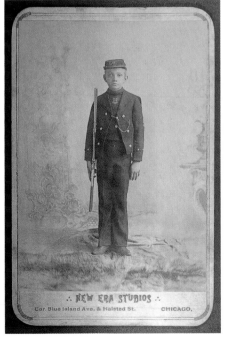

Cabinet card image, circa 1899. The boy in this photo wears a Navy-type blouse and jacket. His kepi has the letters "AG" on the front, and he holds a Helperine B.B. gun. The image is by New Era Studios, Cor. Blue Ave & Halstead St., Chicago. *Courtesy Michael J. Bremer*

An unusual cabinet card of a boy in a Dewey Suit and kepi taken outdoors.

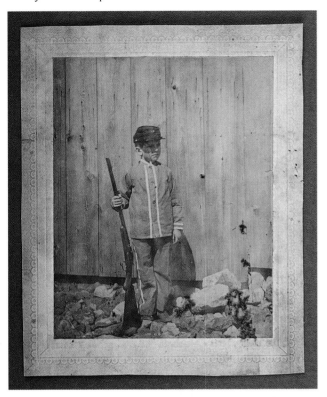

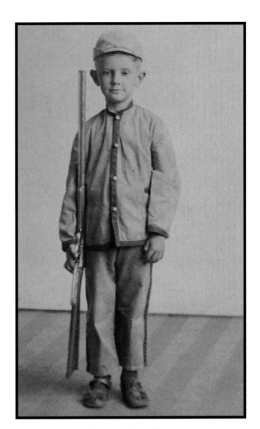

A variation of a Dewey Suit that was probably made at home.

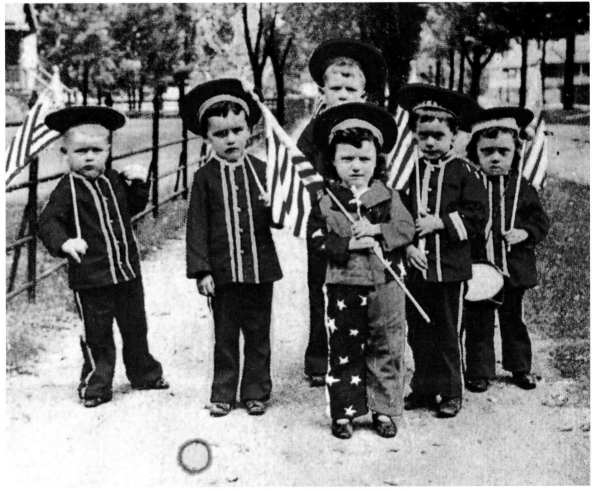

Copyrighted in 1898 by T.W. Ingersoll, this hand-colored stereo view is entitled "Brave Boys in Blue Starting for Manila."

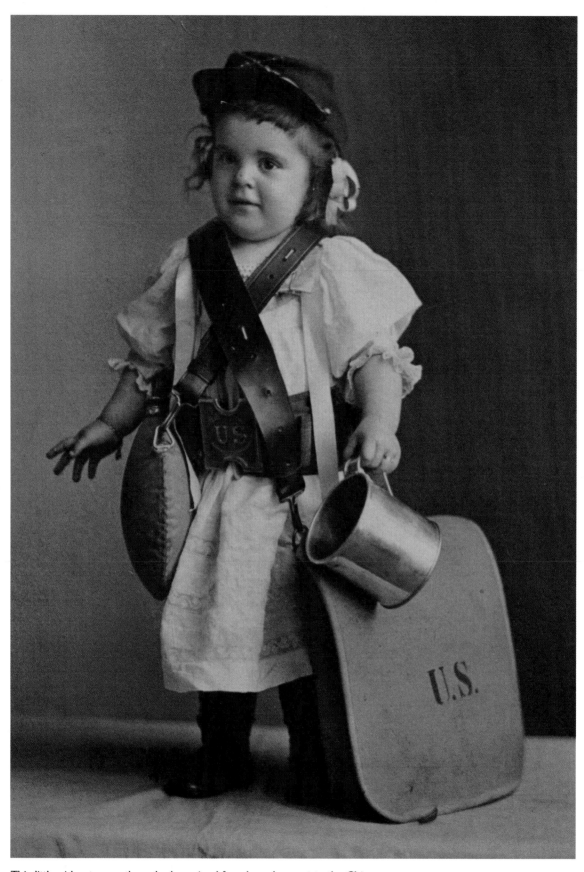

This little girl got more than she bargained for when she went to the Chicago photographer who took this photograph. The gear she wears is Spanish-American War surplus, probably on hand as props in the studio. *Courtesy Terri Stewart*

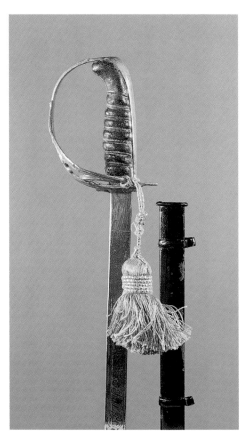

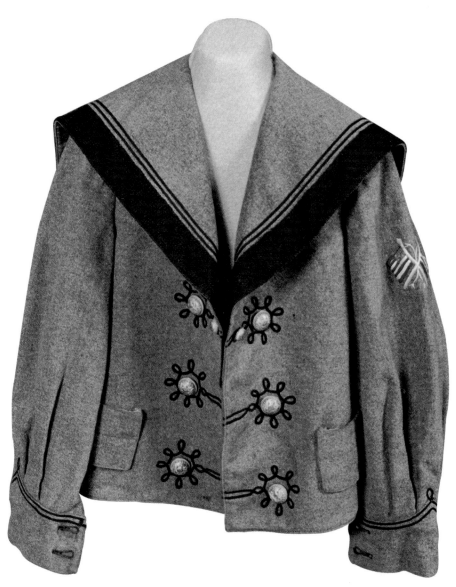

A German-made early-20th-century boy's sword has a lightly etched blade mounted backward with the fuller on the wrong side. The etching shows a scene of two knights jousting before a castle and tents. The ricasso has a mark composed of a seated king with a sword over the words "SMF/WAFFEN-/ABTEILUNG/ SOLINGEN" (the mark of Stoker & Cie). The cast hilt shows the least possible attention to detail. *Courtesy Man at Arms Magazine*

The beautiful handmade wool Navy-inspired bib jacket, circa 1900, is fully lined and has direct-embroidered crossed flags on the shoulder and quatrefoil around the large buttons that serve as decoration. The two smaller buttons on the front are for a small chain, which serves as the closure for the jacket.

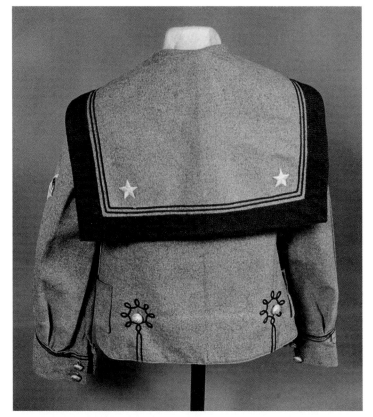

Back of the bib jacket.

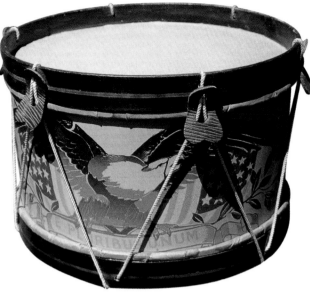

A period child's drum featuring a patriotic theme. *Courtesy Noble & Cooley Co.*

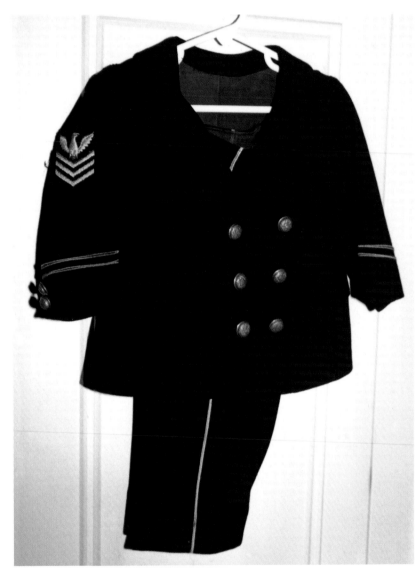

A high-quality, ready-to-wear Navy-styled coat and trousers. The coat features officer-style Spanish-American War-era buttons. *Courtesy Kathleen MacDonald Collection*

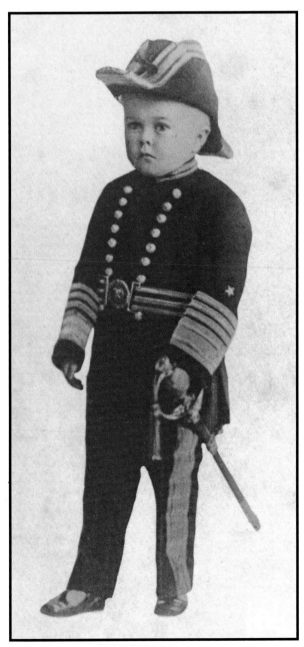

Admiral Dewey remained a hero in American culture long after the Spanish-American War ended. This child, dressed as a "Dewey Figure," wears an exquisite Navy admiral ensemble. The fore-and-aft cap, Navy belt, and sword may indeed be the real thing, scaled to fit this youngster.

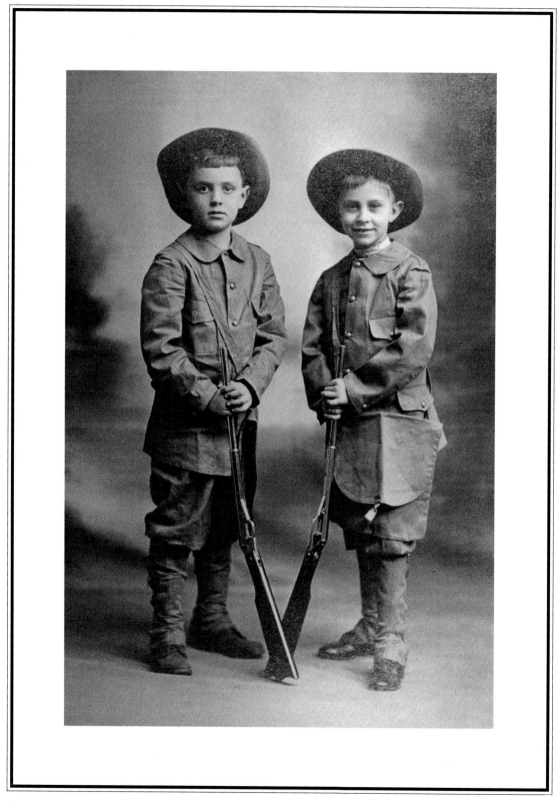

This McCormick Studio, Quincy, Illinois, photo features two boys dressed as Spanish-American War soldiers preparing for battle. *Courtesy Michael J. Bremer*

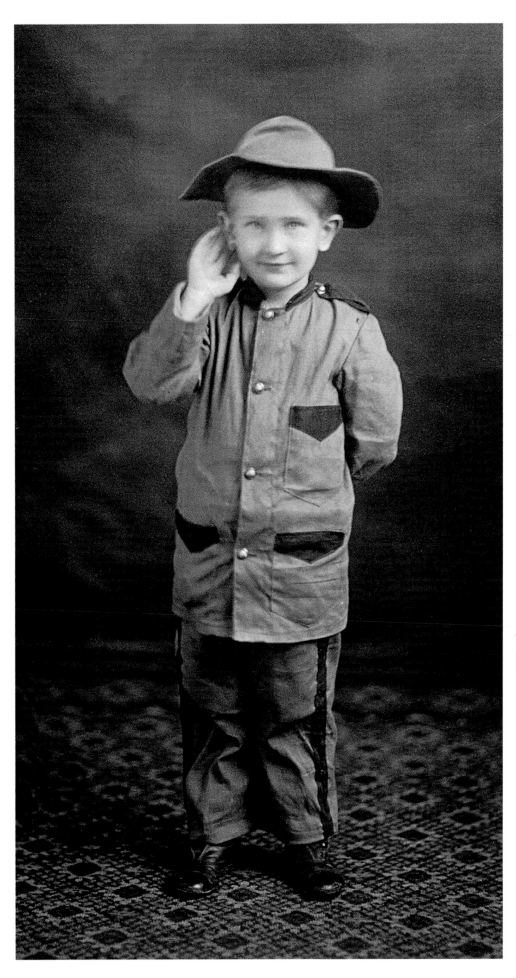

This little Rough Rider listens for the sound of the call that will take him to battle at San Juan Hill.

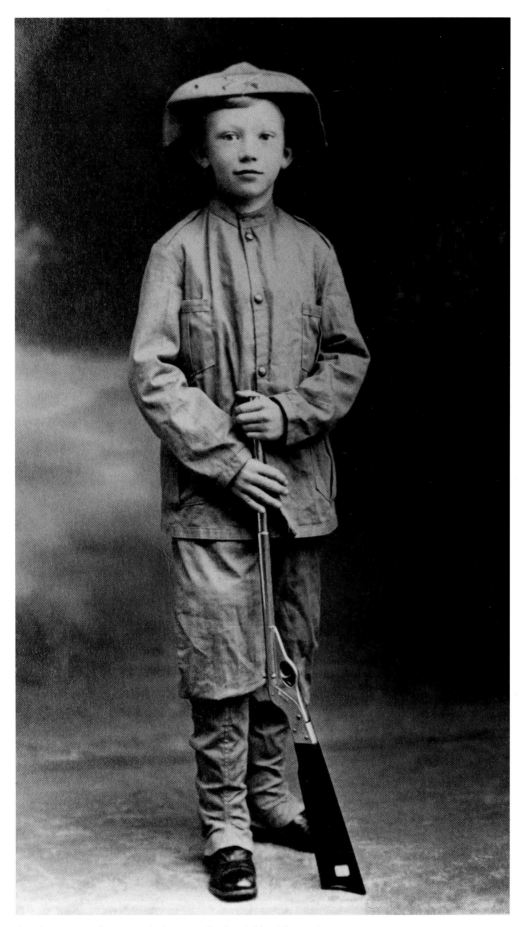

Another outstanding period photograph of a child soldier with every
detail in place. *Courtesy Herb Peck*

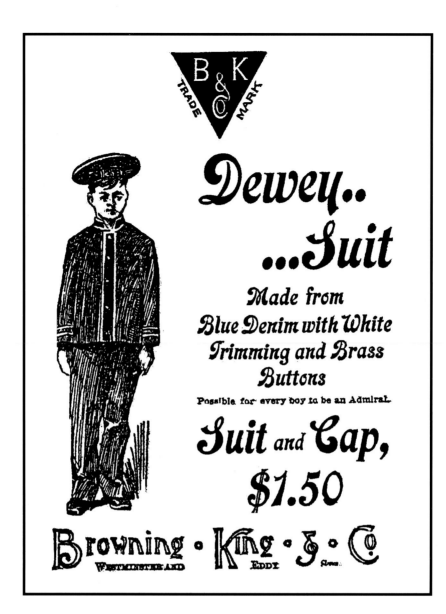

A terrific commercially produced postcard of a child dressed in a Teddy Roosevelt Rough Rider costume in three different poses. Everything is perfect, from his campaign hat and the kerchief around his neck to his cartridge belt and small sidearm.

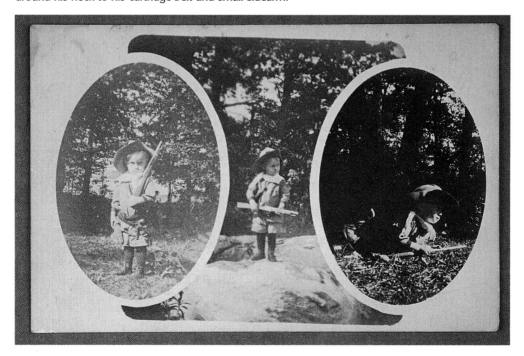

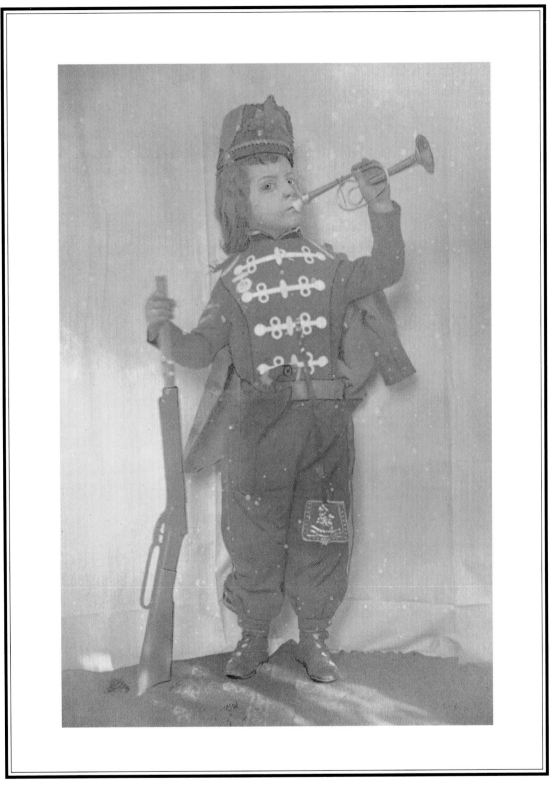

By all estimates, this image of an unusual bugle boy probably dates between 1896 to1903, determined primarily by the model of Heilprin cast-iron B.B. gun. The delightful *chasseur*-style outfit he wears is pure fantasy.

A New Century ───────────

A boy characterized as a sailor appears in this postcard dated December 15, 1915.

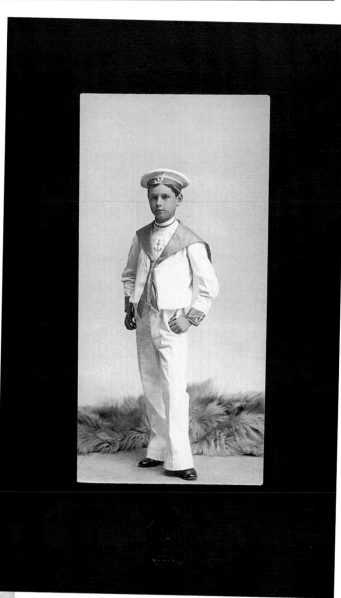

At first glance the sailor suit and format of this Victorian-period cabinet card has a decidedly European feel. Closer inspection reveals the G.M. Bolton, Rockville, Connecticut, studio stamp in the frame.

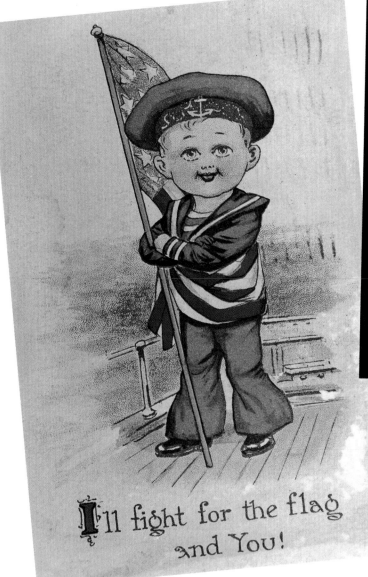

I'll fight for the flag and You!

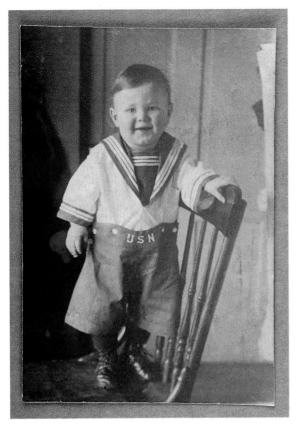

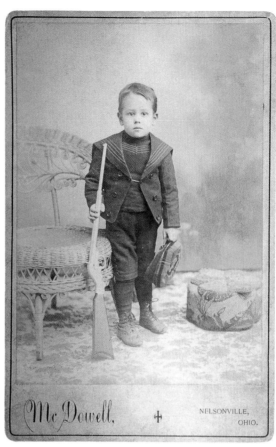

A boy in a naval-type blouse and jacket holding a kepi and 4th model (20th century) Daisy B.B. gun, circa 1900 to 1903. The cabinet card image is by McDowell, Nelsonville, Ohio. *Courtesy Michael J. Bremer*

McDowell,   NELSONVILLE, OHIO.

A happy toddler in a U.S. Navy-inspired jumpsuit.

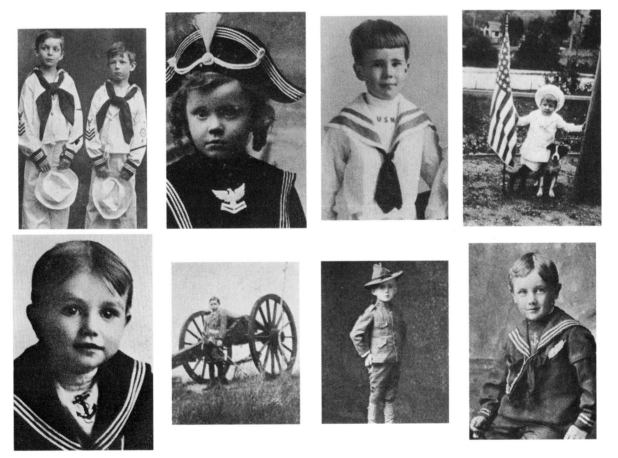

The images of the boys in this series of photos come from the Naval Academy yearbook "Lucky Bag" during the years 1921, 1922, and 1923. Seniors included a photo of themselves as children on the page with their graduation photos. Many boys of this era who attended military academies came from families with a long tradition of military service. *Courtesy National Museum of Naval Aviation Archives, Pensacola, Florida*

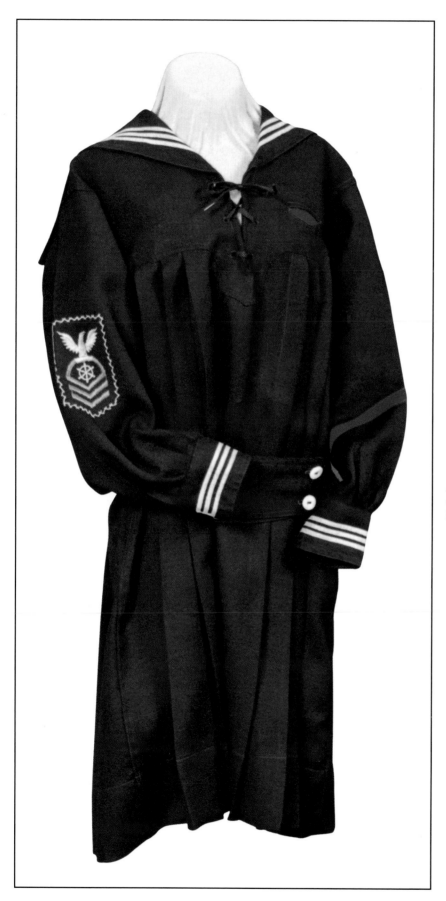

A girl's wool dress similar to the ones offered (right) by Sears Roebuck in the fall of 1916.

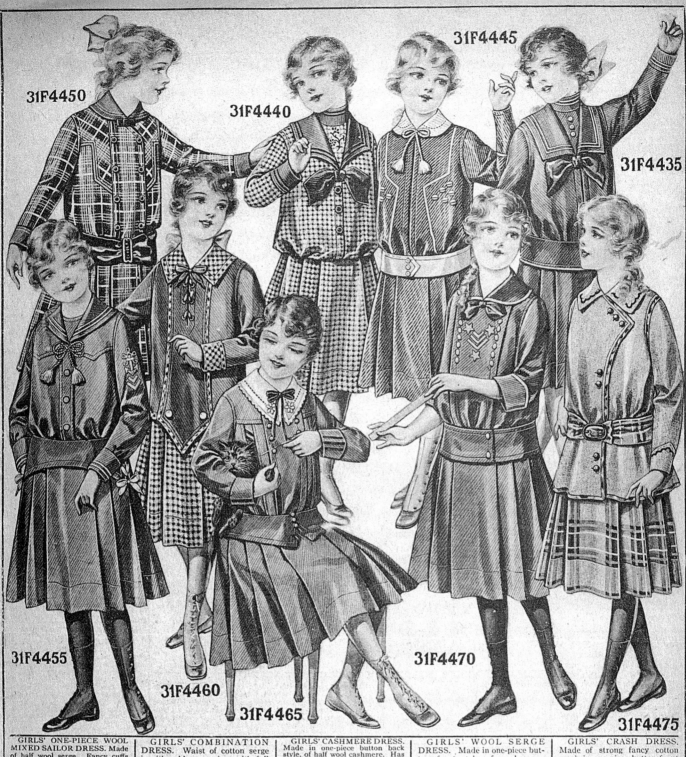

31F4450

31F4440

31F4445

31F4435

31F4455

31F4460

31F4465

31F4470

31F4475

GIRLS' ONE-PIECE WOOL MIXED SAILOR DRESS. Made of half wool serge. Fancy cuffs and neat sailor collar trimmed with red braid and finished with red cord tie. Buttons visibly in front with fancy buttons. Has middy effect belt, stitched at top only, and red silk lacing at sides. Skirt is full plaited. State age. Average shipping weight, 1¾ lbs.

No. **31F4455**
Navy blue.
No. **31F4456** EACH
Wine. **$2.98**

GIRLS' PLAID COTTON SUITING DRESS. Made in one-piece button front style. Has neat collar and cuffs of solid color suiting, and loose belt of velveteen finished with buckle in front. Full plaited skirt. A serviceable school dress. **State age.** Av. shpg. wt., 1½ lbs.

No. **31F4450**
Wine. EACH
No. **31F4451**
Green. **$1.00**

GIRLS' COMBINATION DRESS. Waist of cotton serge in either blue or wine, with full plaited skirt and trimmings of cotton woven shepherd check suiting. Has neat lacing in front and trimming buttons of red. A pleasing combination, as well as serviceable. **State age.** Average shipping weight, 1¼ pounds.

No. **31F4460**
Blue.
No. **31F4461** EACH
Wine. **$1.33**

GIRLS' TWO-PIECE SAILOR DRESS. Made of woven shepherd check cotton suiting. Sailor collar and cuffs of red rep are trimmed with soutache braid. Has black bow tie. Has sewed on embroidered dickey of shepherd check with high collar of red rep to match sailor collar. Full plaited skirt is attached to cambric underwaist. **State age.** Average shipping weight, 1½ pounds.

No. **31F4440** EACH
Shepherd check. **$1.48**

GIRLS' CASHMERE DRESS. Made in one-piece button back style, of half wool cashmere. Has collar of embroidered and hemstitched lawn, finished with neat velveteen tie. Fancy waist and turnback cuffs trimmed with straps of velveteen. Wide belt is stitched at top only. Skirt is full plaited. **State age.** Average shipping weight, 1¼ pounds.

No. **31F4465**
Navy blue.
No. **31F4466**
Wine.
No. **31F4467** EACH
Brown. **$2.98**

GIRLS' ONE-PIECE SUITING DRESS. Made of fancy cotton suiting, neatly embroidered in two-tone silk. Has up to date cuffs. Collar of hemstitched pique. Skirt full plaited. Blue dress has belt and piping of tan. Wine dress is trimmed with green. Buttons invisibly in front. **State age.** Average shipping weight, 1¾ pounds.

No. **31F4445**
Blue.
No. **31F4446** EACH
Wine. **$1.55**

GIRLS' WOOL SERGE DRESS. Made in one-piece button front style of wool serge. Waist is neatly embroidered in front and trimmed with fancy buttons. Collar and turnback cuffs piped in red. Buttons invisibly in front. Skirt is full plaited. **State age.** Average shipping weight, 1¾ pounds.

No. **31F4470**
Navy blue.
No. **31F4471** EACH
Brown. **$3.79**

GIRLS' COTTON SERGE DRESS. Made of good cotton serge in the standard sailor style, buttoning invisibly in front. The sailor collar, also the high neck collar and cuffs, are trimmed with two rows of red braid. Has large bow tie of rep. Belt stitched at top only, giving it the middy effect. Skirt full plaited. **State age.** Average shpg. weight, 1½ lbs.

No. **31F4435** EACH
Navy blue. **$1.29**

GIRLS' CRASH DRESS. Made of strong fancy cotton crash in one-piece button front style. Waist is cut in coat effect, giving it the appearance of a two-piece dress. Has loose belt of plaid, finished with buckle. Skirt of neat pattern plaid, full plaited. Average shpg. wt., 1½ pounds.

No. **31F4475**
Blue.
No. **31F4476** EACH
Tan. **$1.76**

Girls' Dresses on this page are furnished in sizes 6 to 14 years. **Be sure to state size when ordering.**

Age, years.	6	8	10	12	14
Average bust measure, in.	28	29	30	32	34
Average length, in.	26	28	32	38	42

☞ **If Parcel Post Shipment Include Amount of Charges Extra. See Page 755.**

Sig. 3—Chi.

SEARS, ROEBUCK AND CO. 150F CHICAGO, ILL.

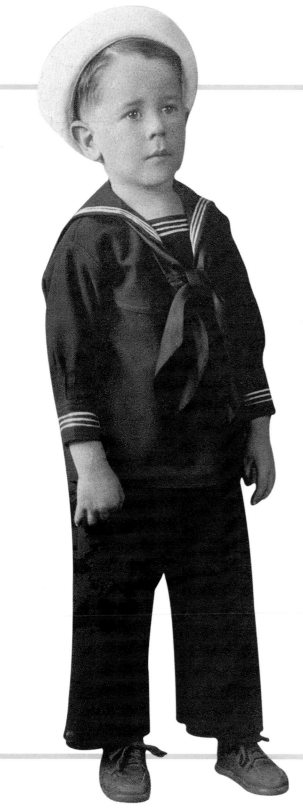

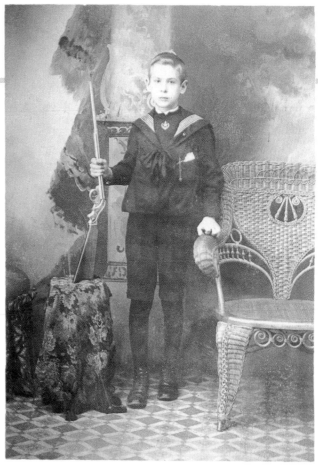

An image with many elements that include a 4th model or 20th-century Daisy B.B. gun, circa 1900 to1903. *Courtesy Michael J. Bremer.*

A melancholy soldier guards his backyard.

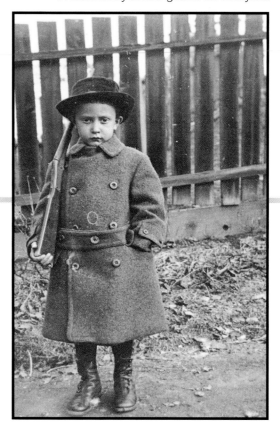

Whereas there is nothing unusual about the sailor suit, what is of note in this photograph is the white cap. Images of this era of boys in sailor suits usually include the navy-blue "flat cap." White caps are generally not seen on children until much later.

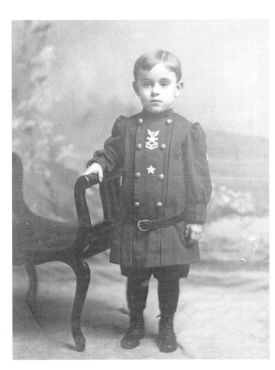

A tunic with leatherette Sam Browne belt and military-style buttons. *Courtesy Kathleen MacDonald Collection*

A beautiful Navy-inspired blouse with appliqued insignia.

Fashionable suits that suggest military influence. *Courtesy Sears Graphics*

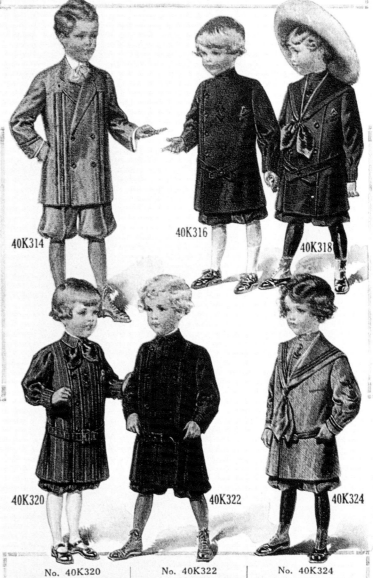

Ucanttear BRAND SUITS FOR LITTLE FELLOWS

No. 40K314
$3.35 PRETTY BROWN AND GRAY MIXTURE SUIT of good weight all wool cassimere. Coat has yoke effect, plaits trimmed with tape, slash pockets, derby back, bottom facings and English twill lining. Knickerbocker pants with side pockets, one hip pocket and strap and buckle at knee. SIZES—5 to 9 years. State boy's age.

No. 40K316
$1.75 LITTLE FEL-LOWS' MILITARY COLLAR RUSSIAN SUIT of good weight soft finish wool and cotton mixed Union cassimere. Coat is trimmed with black tape and silk embroidered emblem. Silk handkerchief effect in breast pocket, and belt of same material. Bloomer pants with elastic bottoms, full lining and taped seams. SIZES—2½ to 6 years. State boy's age.

No. 40K318
$1.90 BLUE RUSSIAN BLOUSE SUIT of good weight soft finish wool and cotton mixed cassimere. Sailor collar trimmed with soutache. Detachable shield, silk handkerchief effect in breast pocket, silk tie, and belt of same material. Bloomer pants with elastic bottoms; double stitched and taped seams. SIZES—2½ to 6 years. State boy's age.

No. 40K320
$2.50 ETON RUSSIAN BLOUSE SUIT in bluish gray all wool material. Coat buttons on the side and has silk embroidered emblem, silk handkerchief effect in breast pocket, black tie, and belt of same material. Bloomer pants have side pockets, one hip pocket and elastic bottoms. SIZES—2½ to 6 years. State boy's age.

No. 40K322
$2.75 LITTLE FEL-LOWS' SUIT in popular Eton Russian style. Made of excellent quality cotton worsted. Coat collar trimmed with brown tape, leather lined belt, cuff effect and ivory buttons. Bloomer pants with double stitched and taped seams, side pockets, one hip pocket and elastic bottoms. SIZES—4 to 8 years. State boy's age.

No. 40K324
$3.75 VERY DRESSY SUIT of medium weight all wool cassimere, in gray mixture with light blue trimmings. Coat has gray silk tie, silk embroidered emblem on left sleeve, leather belt and fancy trimmed cuffs made to button. Bloomer pants with elastic bottoms. Finely tailored. SIZES—2½ to 6 years. Mention boy's age.

ILLUSTRATIONS SHOW GARMENTS IN THEIR ACTUAL STYLES AND COLORS. Note descriptions for sizes, and when ordering state boy's age and whether he is large, small or average size. Average shipping weight of suits on this page, each, 2¼ pounds.

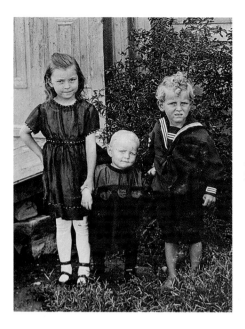

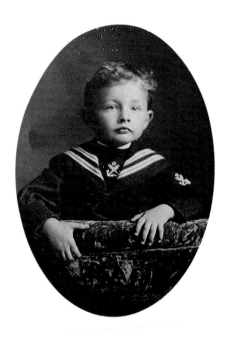

A summer sailor out in the yard with his two sisters.

Yet another portrait of a boy in a sailor suit. This format and fashion style were standards for the post-Spanish-American War era right through WW I.

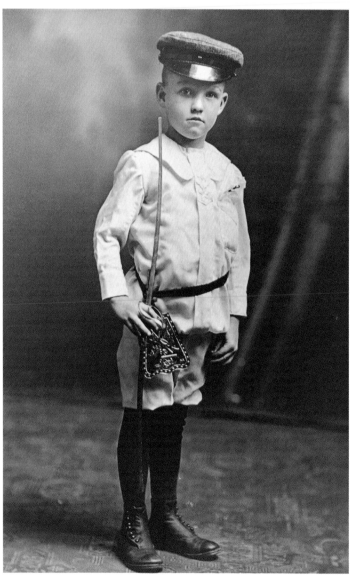

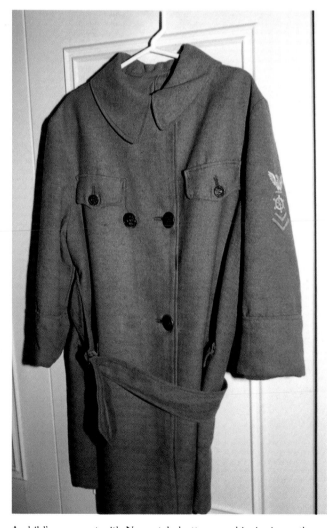

A typical summer linen outfit with an added appliqued Navy insignia in the middle of the chest. The subject holds an unidentified boy's saber with decorative sabertash.

A child's overcoat with Navy-style buttons and insignia on the sleeve. *Courtesy Kathleen MacDonald Collection*

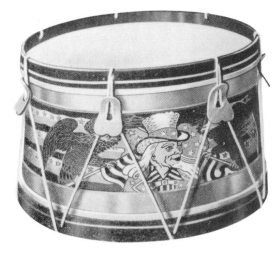

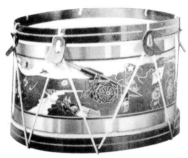

A selection from the Noble & Cooley 1912 catalog (right), which features Uncle Sam on a metal shell, then and now. *Courtesy Noble & Cooley Co.*

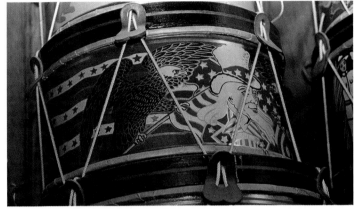

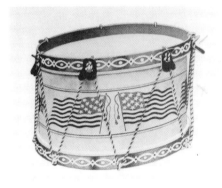

Two selections (above and right) from the Noble & Cooley 1910 catalog. *Courtesy Noble & Cooley Co.*

A wooden shell drum features Civil War soldiers from the 1910 Noble & Cooley catalog. *Courtesy Noble & Cooley Co.*

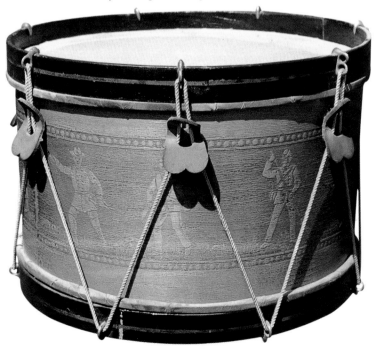

A post-Victorian cabinet card image of two children in beautiful attire. The boy wears a sailor suit similar in style to the selections offered by Sears Roebuck Co. in the spring of 1914 (opposite page).

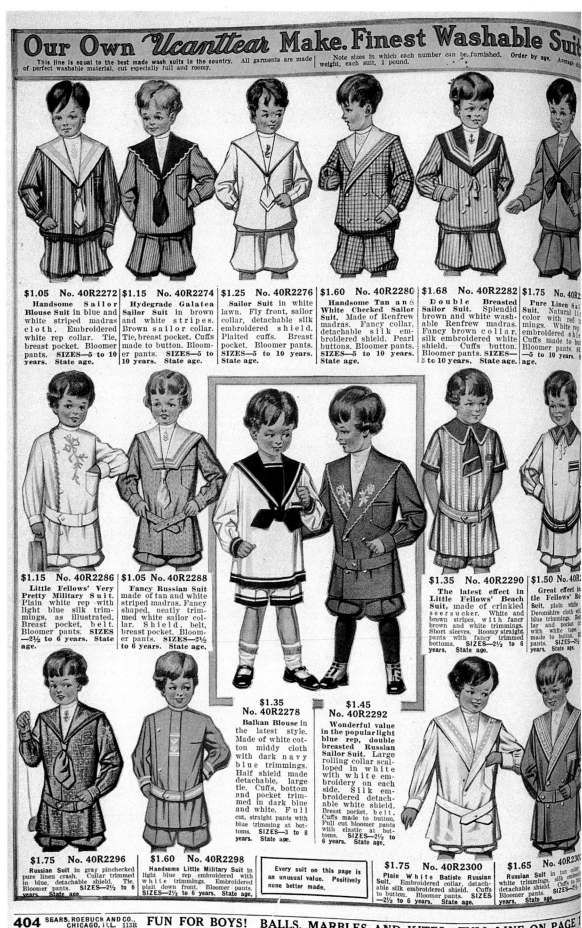

Courtesy Sears Graphics

66

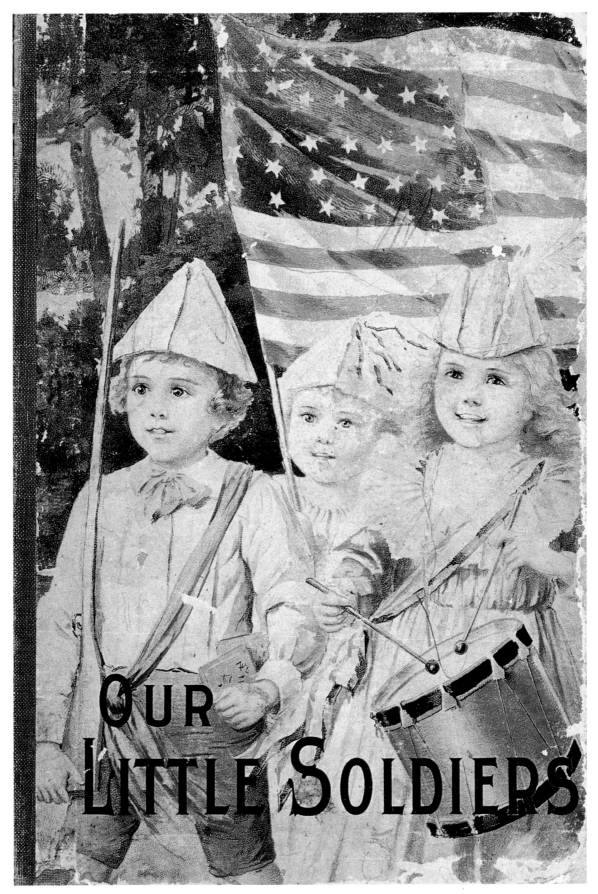

Our Little Soldiers: No publishing date or copyright appears in this book, but an inscription from Christmas 1906 gives a clue to its age. The inside cover reads: "Amusing Tales of Animals and Pets, Glowing Scenes in Fairyland; Outdoor and Indoor Sports; Fireside Poems Etc.; The Whole Affording Many Happy Hours to the Young." It was compiled and edited by Alice Huntington, superbly embellished with many choice illustrations, and issued by Juvenile Publishers.

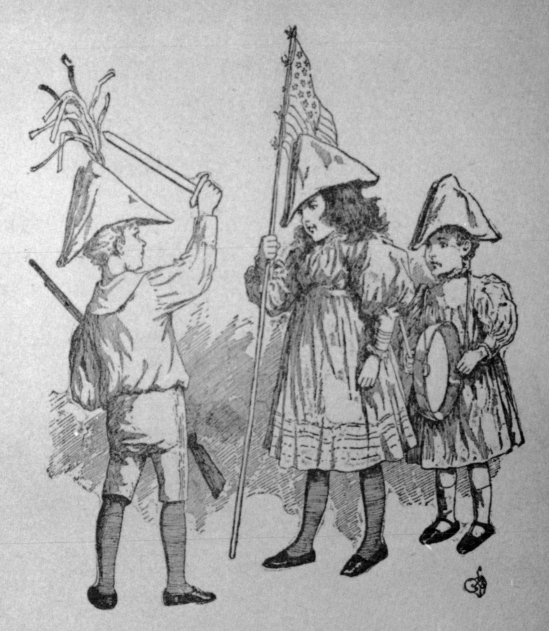

Rub-a-dub-dub! The pattering rain
Beats aloud on the window-pane.
  Who cares for that? With a paper hat,
  A stick and a pan and a rat-tat-tat,
In rain or in shine, sword, banner, and drum,
  The soldiers come!

MARGARET JOHNSON.

The Little Soldier

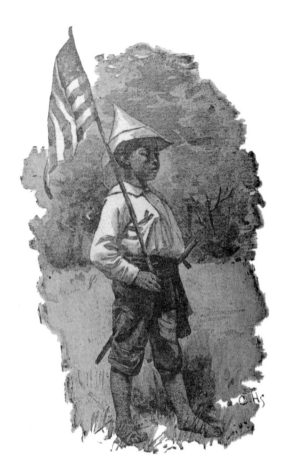

"Oh I would be a soldier boy!"
Said little Sammy Black.
"I'd have a gun and march along,
A knapsack on my back!"

I'd never be a coward, no!
I'd never turn and run;
I'd stand right up before the foe
And shoot them with my gun."

Then Sammy got a wooden sword,
A crimson belt he wore;
A banner too, of red and blue,
Above he bravely bore.

And when he got outside the gate
Some turkeys there he met;
"I'll scatter them," brave Sammy said;
"I'll make them fly, I'll bet!"

The gobblers saw the crimson belt,
And then prepared to fight;
And on the boy, with flapping wings,
They straightaway did alight.

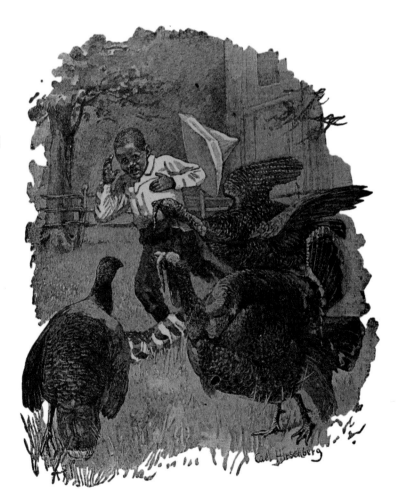

The turkeys screamed "Ca boodle boo!
Ka wee! Ka wee! Ka wee!"
And with a flap the paper cap
Was split in two or three.

"Oh help! Oh my!" the soldier cried;
Oh help! Oh my! Boo hoo!
Come help me out! Oh mamma come!
I don't know what to do!"

His mother came, and with a broom
She put the birds to flight;
But, ah, alas! The soldier boy
Was in a sorry plight.

Then with a quaver Sammy said,
"Such fighters I despise;
'Twas two to one, and then you see,
They took me by surprise."

—H. Elliott McBride

69

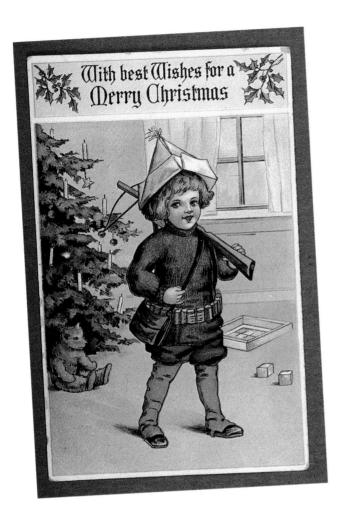

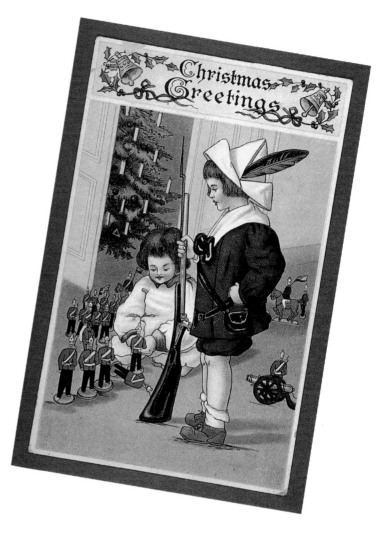

Four Christmas cards from England and America
with children in a military theme.

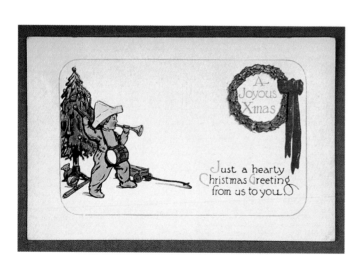

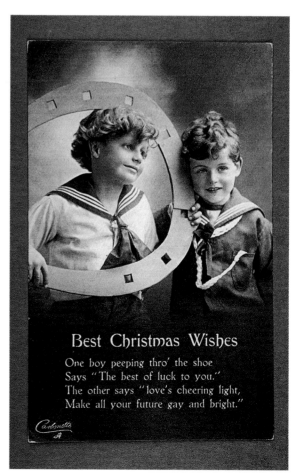

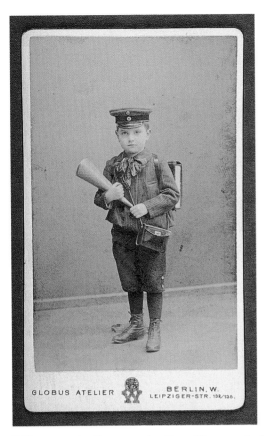

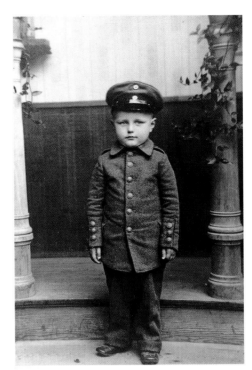

An Imperial-era German child in a 1910 model tunic.

Circa 1902 image of a German schoolboy. The cone he holds is filled with candies and treats. The German tradition of giving goody-filled cornucopias is followed so children won't cry when they leave home for their first day of school.

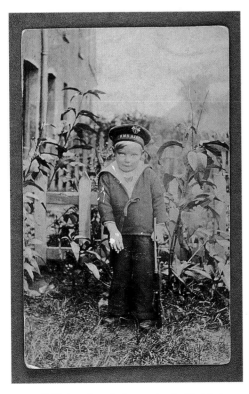

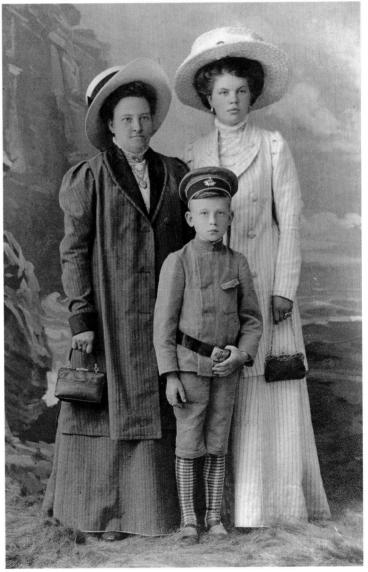

A very young British sailor photographed with his toy gun on a postcard format image. His cap tally reads: "H.M.S. AJAX."

This boy wears a highly stylized German field-officer's uniform that appears to be homemade.

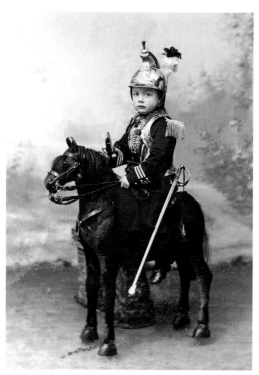

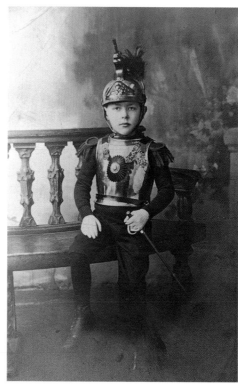

Three closely styled French *cuirassier* breastplates, helmets, and swords (left and opposite page).

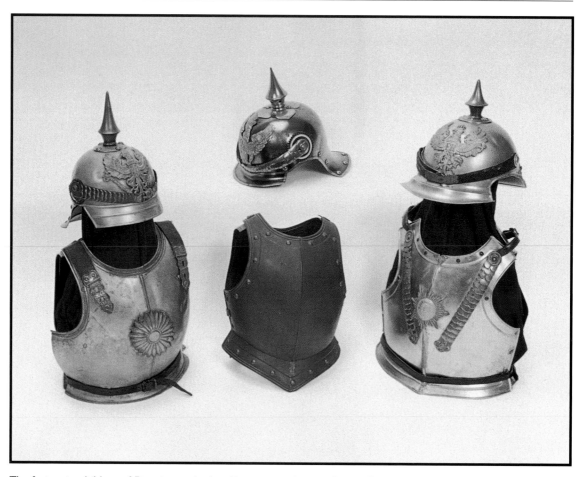

The fortunate children of Prussian and other European *cuirrasier* (heavy Cavalry) officers and NCOs (non-commissioned officers) wore toy "lobster tails," steel helmets, and breastplate armor in the 19th and early-20th century. These outfits emulated the impressive mounted armor worn during parade-dress occasions by their fathers. These children's outfits (shown) were produced to accommodate boys three to five years old. The left and right helmets are of 1860s Prussian design, as is the breastplate on the right. The left breastplate is probably Austrian or Italian, while the center is Victorian British. The center helmet is Jaeger zu Pferde of 1890s vintage. *Courtesy Marie DiMartini Whittmann Collection. Photo: Charles Jenkins, III*

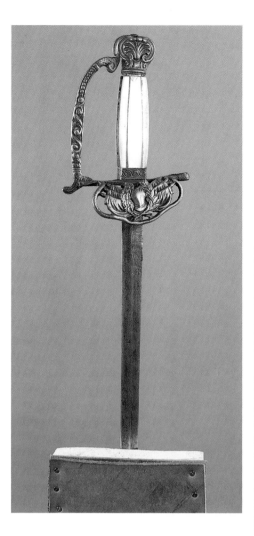

French-pattern boy's small sword of mediocre quality, which does, however, feature mother-of-pearl slab grips. *Courtesy Man at Arms Magazine*

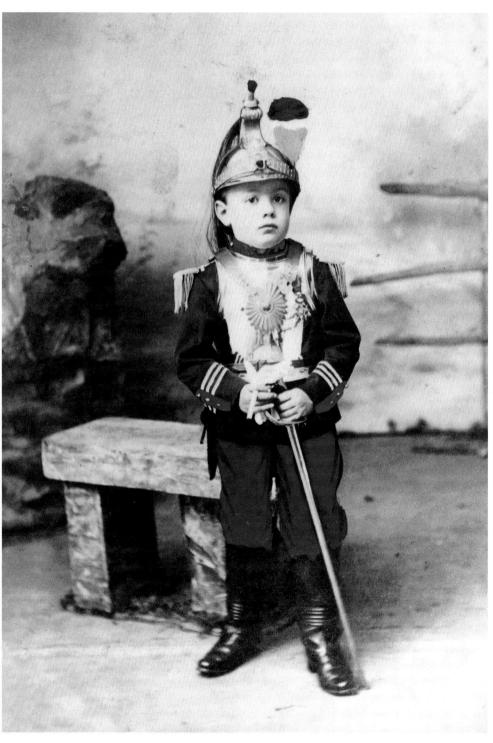

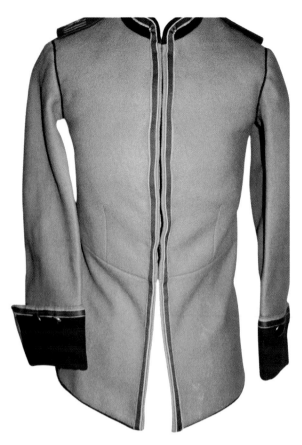
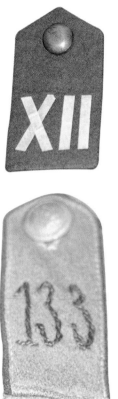
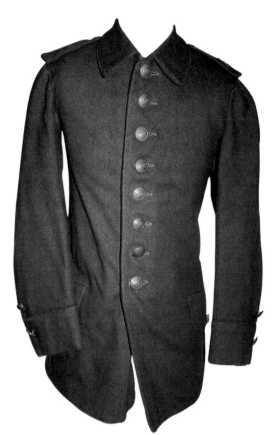

German Imperial tunic. *Courtesy Peter Coleman*

Imperial Bavarian tunic with round crown buttons.
Courtesy Peter Coleman

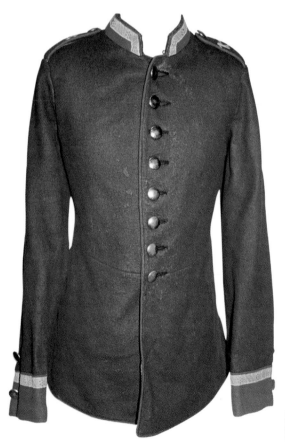
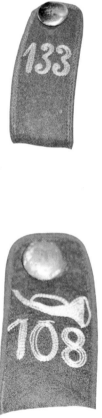
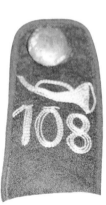
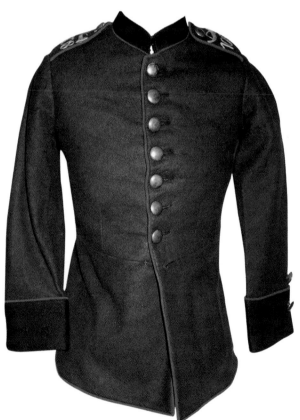

Prussian Infantry tunic. *Courtesy Peter Coleman*

Jäeger Unit tunic. *Courtesy Peter Coleman*

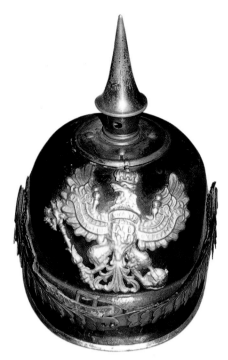

Prussian enlisted-lineman's helmet.
Courtesy Peter Coleman

Beautifully tailored British officer child's outfit is shown placed upon a miniature heavily carved child's corner chair. The diminutive Victorian outfit is sized to fit a two- or three-year-old child. It includes a gold-bullion-decorated red and blue tunic complete with matching gold brocade epaulets and buttons, white riding breeches, brocade cartouche belt, and white cloth sword strap and frog. The outfit is stored in an English officer's metal letterbox (shown). *Courtesy Marie DiMartini Whittmann Collection. Photo: Charles Jenkins, III*

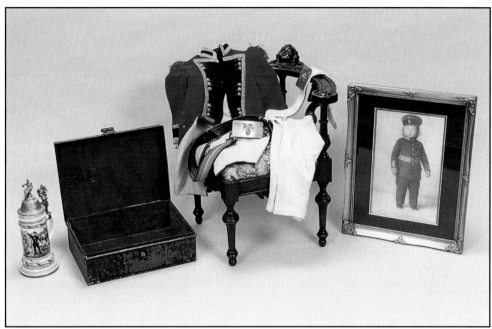

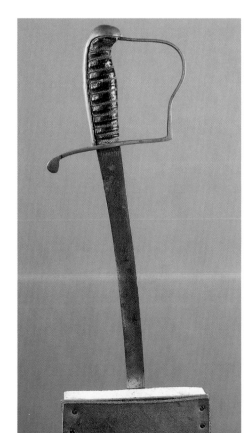

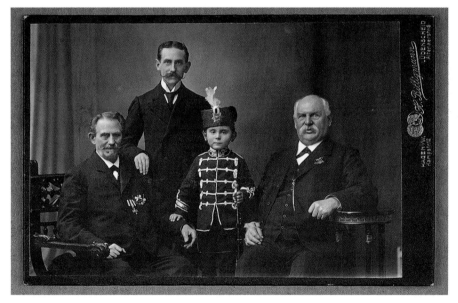

A formal Prussian Hussar Guard-style uniform.

A low-quality boy's saber for a very small child of kindergarten age. *Courtesy Man at Arms Magazine*

"The Great War"

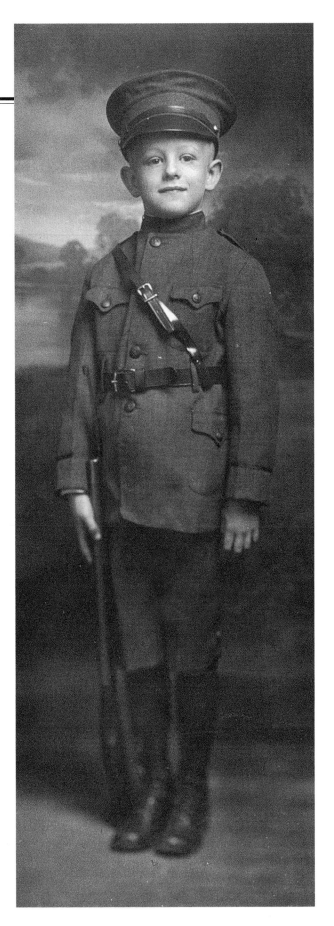

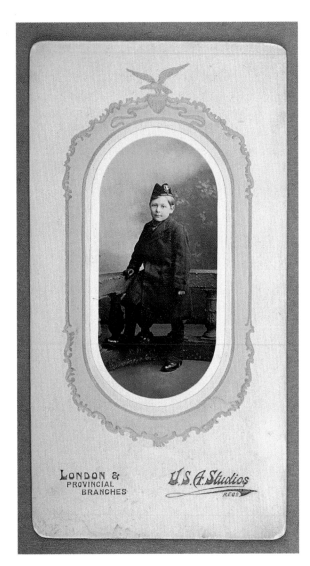

A beautiful cabinet card-format image with a patriotic-style mat of a young Scottish boy. It is unclear whether this photo was taken in the U.S. or England. Note the thistle in his OS cap.

The tip of the bayonet on this soldier's rifle has been clipped and rounded over in an apparent attempt to thwart injury. This highly prized image from the author's collection was photographed in Jackson, Tennessee.

Camp Dix Pictorial Review

Vol. I. No. 7   Camp Dix, N. J., July 20, 1918   Price 10 cents

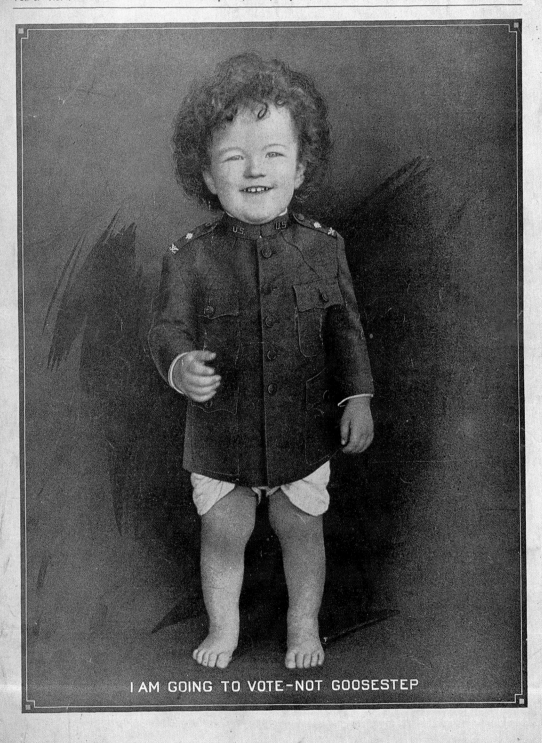

I AM GOING TO VOTE—NOT GOOSESTEP

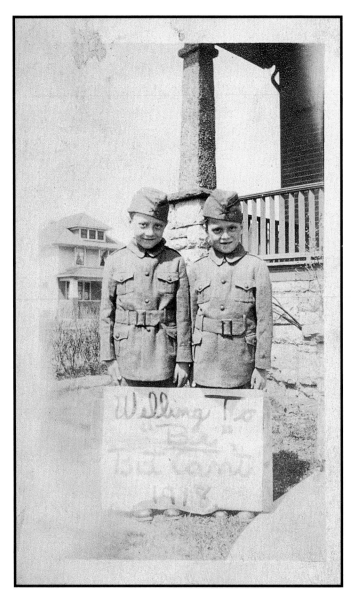

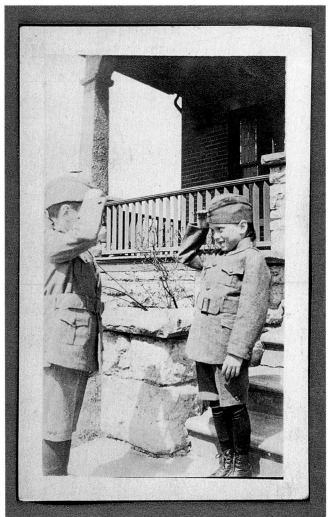

"Willing to be, but can't" says it all for these doughboy twins in 1918.

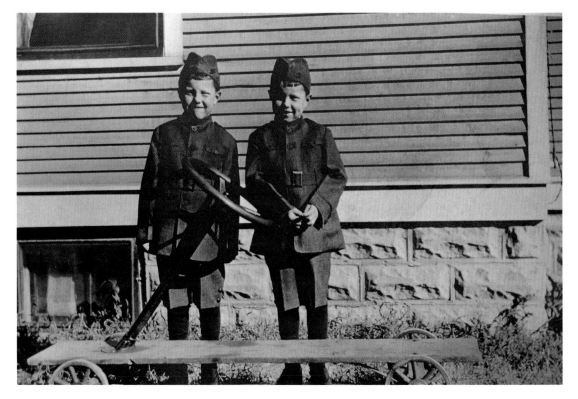

Perfectly pressed and ready for inspection. This set of twins stops for a quick snapshot before heading out on a neighborhood mission in their "scout car." Their mother writes on the reverse of this picture postcard: "I am sending you my soldier boys. They are so proud when they wear their soldier suits, and they want to salute everyone when they have them on."

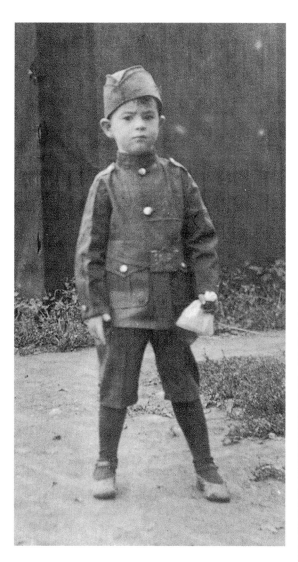

The paper photo-album page under this photo reads, "See my candy. My soldier suit is fine too. I am very brave. I have two sisters."

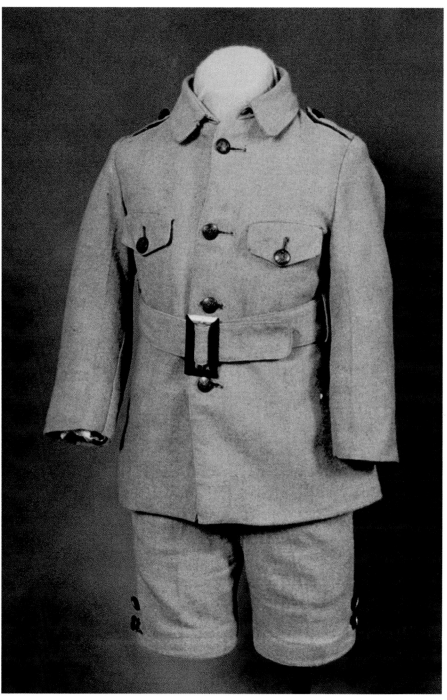

A commercially made WWI Army-style uniform similar to the ones shown on the opposite page.

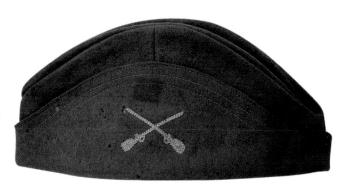

Crossed rifles chain stitched on this early felt OS cap signify Infantry. Crossed cannons would indicate Artillery, crossed sabers signify Cavalry.

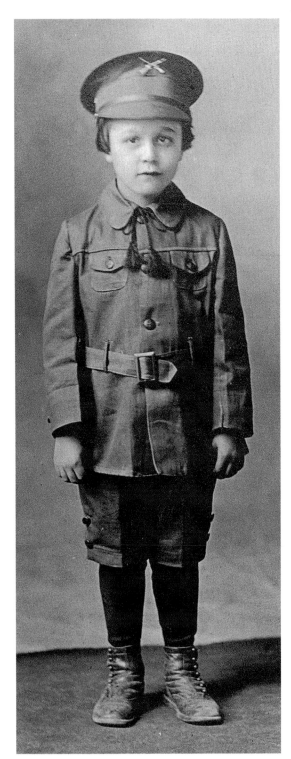

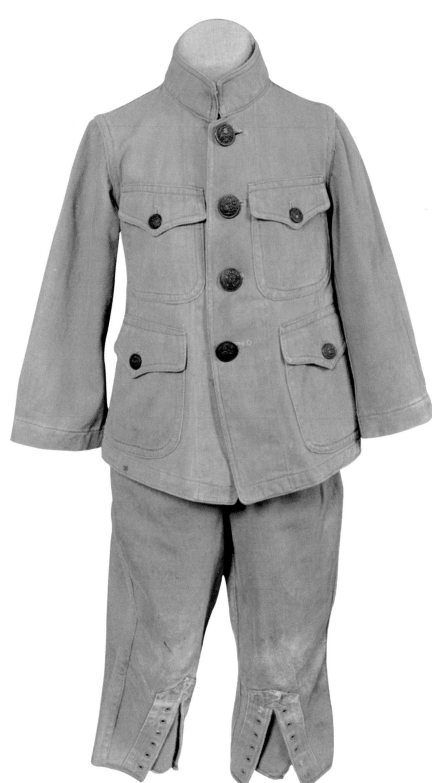

Crossed rifles (like the ones on the young man's hat) signify Infantry.

The trousers for this uniform have lace-up calves, which were covered with leggings. This uniform is for an older boy of about ten or eleven years.

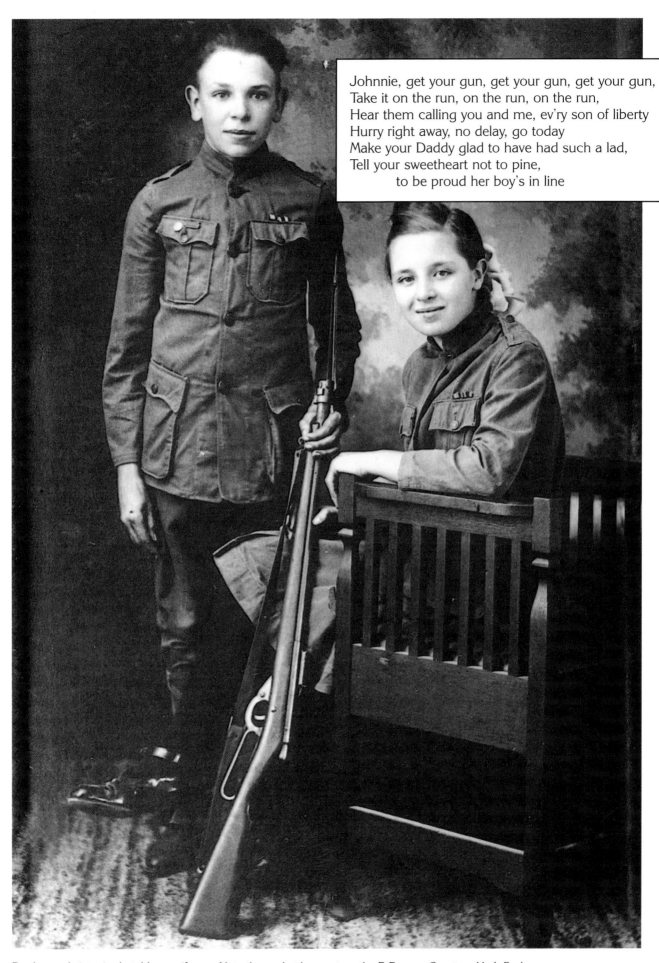

Johnnie, get your gun, get your gun, get your gun,
Take it on the run, on the run, on the run,
Hear them calling you and me, ev'ry son of liberty
Hurry right away, no delay, go today
Make your Daddy glad to have had such a lad,
Tell your sweetheart not to pine,
    to be proud her boy's in line

Brother and sister in doughboy uniforms. Note the socket bayonet on the B.B. gun. *Courtesy Herb Peck*

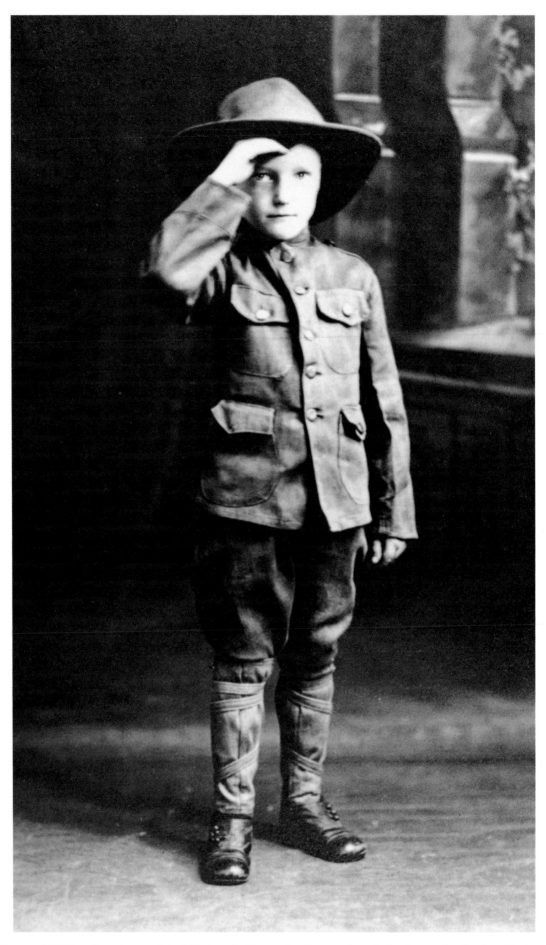

This superb WWI uniform is complete right down to the wool puttees and an obviously oversize Montana Peak campaign hat that may have belonged to a relative.

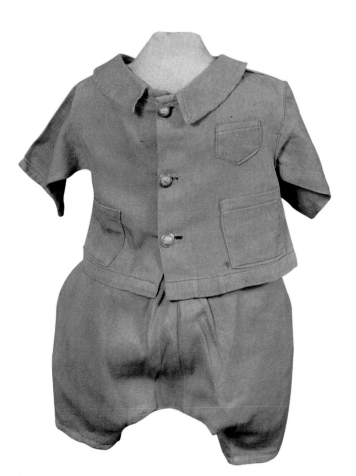

An adorable baby-size doughboy uniform made at home, complete with breeches and Spanish-American War-era tin-back staff buttons.

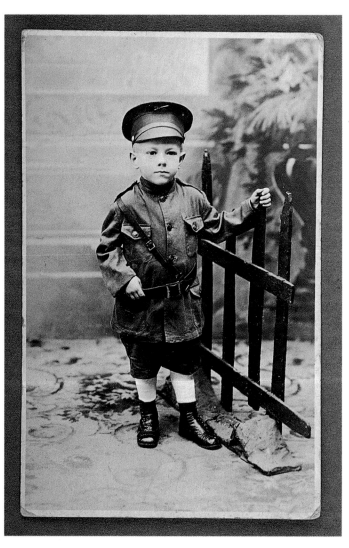

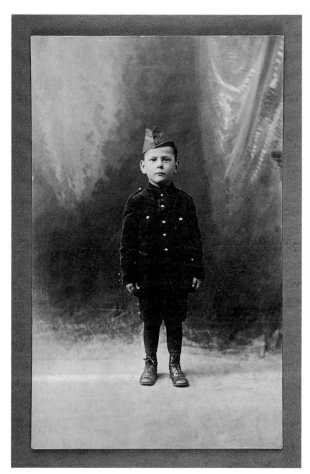

83

Over there over there!
Send the word, send the word
Over there!
That the Yanks are coming,
The drums rum-tumming ev'rywhere!
So prepare, Say a prayer,
Send the word, send the word to beware!
We'll be over, we're coming over,
And we won't come back 'til
It's over Over there!

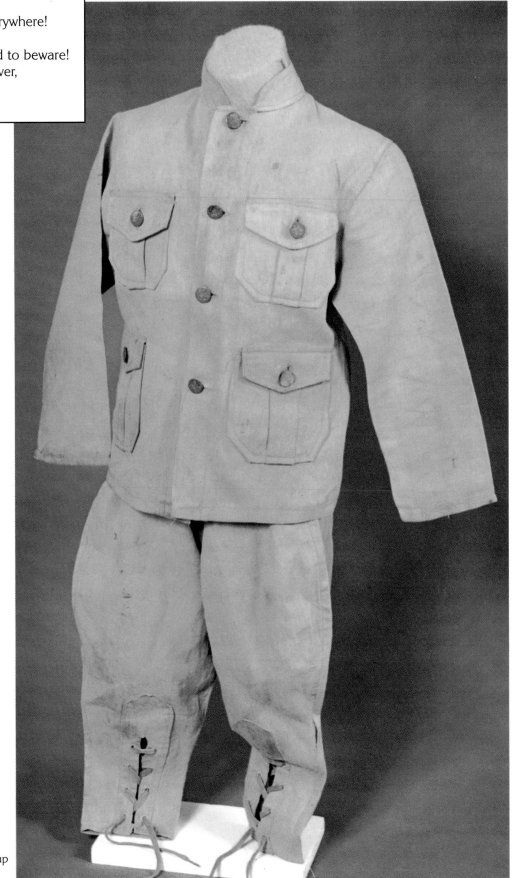

A heavy linen Army tunic and lace-up
breeches with cast buttons.

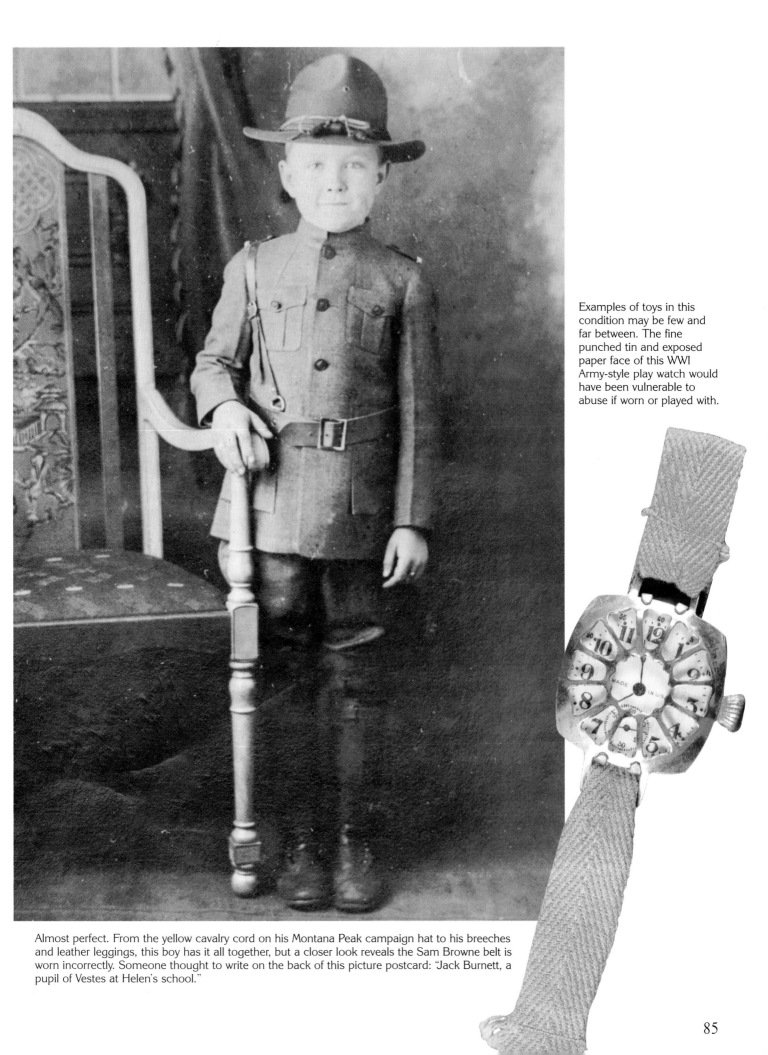

Examples of toys in this condition may be few and far between. The fine punched tin and exposed paper face of this WWI Army-style play watch would have been vulnerable to abuse if worn or played with.

Almost perfect. From the yellow cavalry cord on his Montana Peak campaign hat to his breeches and leather leggings, this boy has it all together, but a closer look reveals the Sam Browne belt is worn incorrectly. Someone thought to write on the back of this picture postcard: "Jack Burnett, a pupil of Vestes at Helen's school."

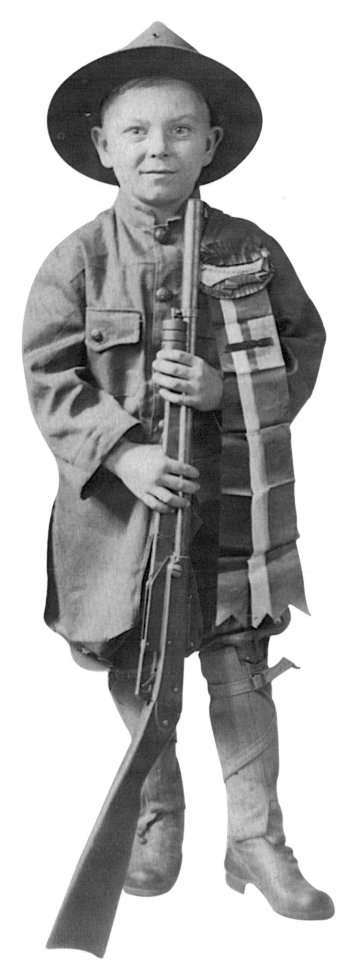

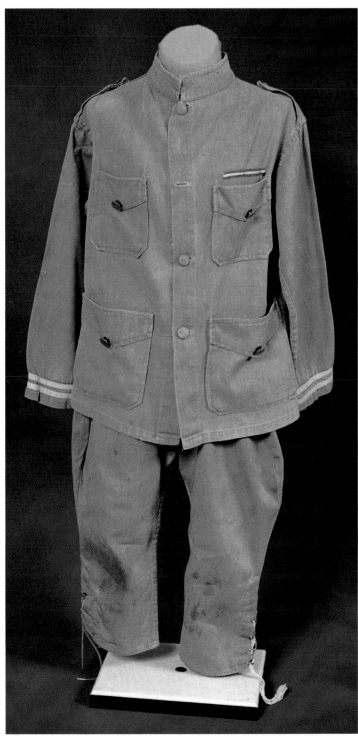

This boy appears to be wearing a small adult-size uniform. His ribbon and B.B. gun are terrifically oversized, making this image highly collectible. Courtesy *Michael J. Bremer*

This doughboy-style uniform was manufactured in the early 1940s during WWII.

Johnnie, get your gun, get your gun, get your gun,
Johnnie show the Hun you're a son of a gun!
Hoist the flag and let her fly,
Yankee Doodle do or die
Pack your little kit, show your grit, do your bit
Yankees to the ranks from the towns and the tanks
Make your mother proud of you
        and the old Red White and Blue

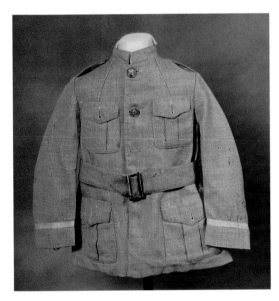

The lightweight wool tunic (above) is missing most of its military-style buttons. The handsome cabinet card image (right) was purchased in a Marietta, Georgia, antiques mall for $10.

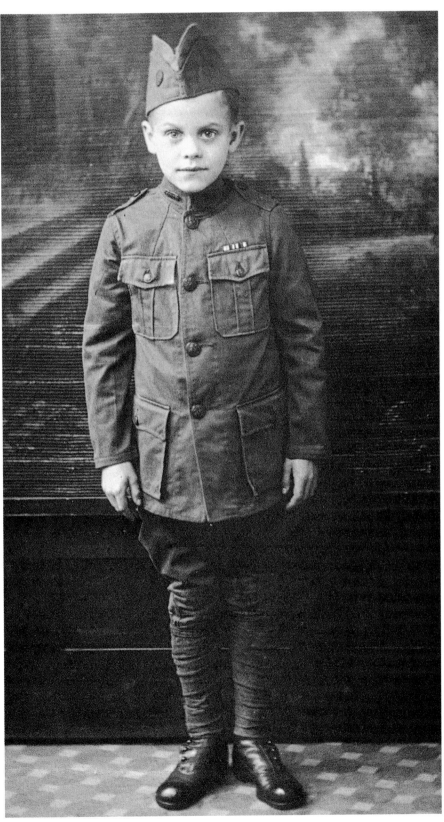

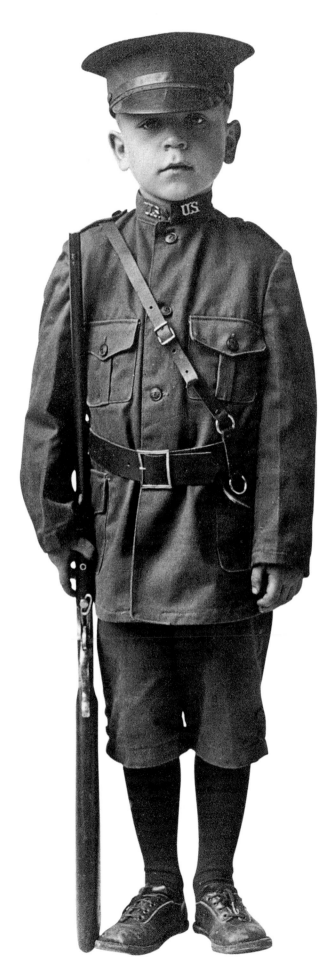

Over there, over there,
Send the word, send the word, over there!
That the Yanks are coming, the Yanks are coming,
The drums rum-tumming ev'ry where
So prepare, say a prayer,
Send the word, send the word to beware
We'll be over, we're coming over,
And we won't come back 'til it's over Over There!

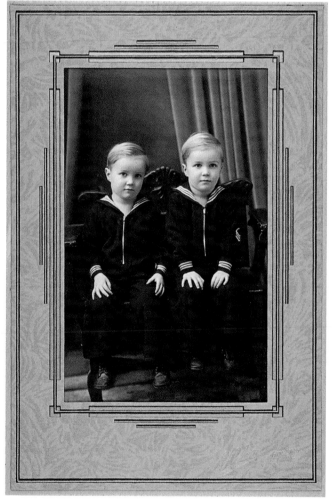

The picture postcard image (left) from Morrow's Studio, Newport, Pennsylvania, is dated 1918. Twin sailors (lower) are ready to ship out in this deco-style mat cabinet card image taken by Holm, Roseau, Minnesota. Sears Roebuck & Company offered "play suits" (right) for the first time in 1918. Among the four selections of military-style costumes was a "Cadet" outfit.

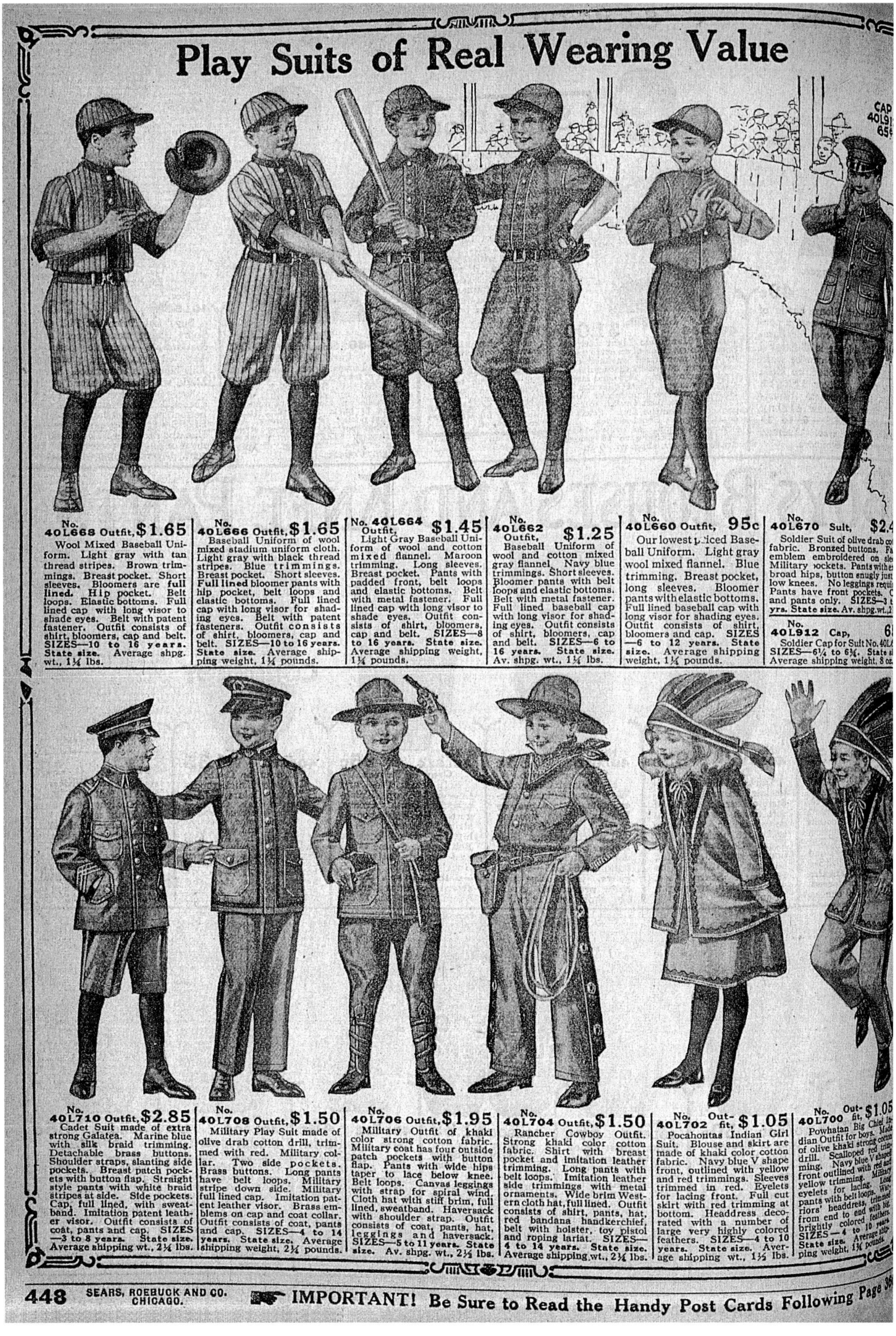

Play Suits of Real Wearing Value

No. 40L668 Outfit, $1.65
Wool Mixed Baseball Uniform. Light gray with tan thread stripes. Brown trimmings. Breast pocket. Short sleeves. Bloomers are **full lined.** Hip pocket. Belt loops. Elastic bottoms. Full lined cap with long visor to shade eyes. Belt with patent fastener. Outfit consists of shirt, bloomers, cap and belt. SIZES—10 to 16 years. **State size.** Average shpg. wt., 1¼ lbs.

No. 40L666 Outfit, $1.65
Baseball Uniform of wool mixed stadium uniform cloth. Light gray with black thread stripes. Blue trimmings. Breast pocket. Short sleeves. **Full lined** bloomer pants with hip pocket, belt loops and elastic bottoms. Full lined cap with long visor for shading eyes. Belt with patent fasteners. Outfit consists of shirt, bloomers, cap and belt. SIZES—10 to 16 years. **State size.** Average shipping weight, 1¼ pounds.

No. 40L664 Outfit, $1.45
Light Gray Baseball Uniform of wool and cotton mixed flannel. Maroon trimming. Long sleeves. Breast pocket. Pants with padded front, belt loops and elastic bottoms. Belt with metal fastener. Full lined cap with long visor to shade eyes. Outfit consists of shirt, bloomers, cap and belt. SIZES—8 to 16 years. **State size.** Average shipping weight, 1¼ pounds.

No. 40L662 Outfit, $1.25
Baseball Uniform of wool and cotton mixed gray flannel. Navy blue trimmings. Short sleeves. Bloomer pants with belt loops and elastic bottoms. Belt with metal fastener. Full lined baseball cap with long visor for shading eyes. Outfit consists of shirt, bloomers, cap and belt. SIZES—6 to 16 years. **State size.** Av. shpg. wt., 1¼ lbs.

No. 40L660 Outfit, 95c
Our lowest priced Baseball Uniform. Light gray wool mixed flannel. Blue trimming. Breast pocket, long sleeves. Bloomer pants with elastic bottoms. Full lined baseball cap with long visor for shading eyes. Outfit consists of shirt, bloomers and cap. SIZES—6 to 12 years. **State size.** Average shipping weight, 1¼ pounds.

No. 40L670 Suit, $2.4
Soldier Suit of olive drab co fabric. Bronzed buttons. F emblem embroidered on sle Military pockets. Pants with e broad hips, button snugly jus low knees. No leggings requi Pants have front pockets. C and pants only. SIZES—3 t yrs. **State size.** Av. shpg. wt., 2

No. 40L912 Cap, 6
Soldier Cap for Suit No. 40L SIZES—6¼ to 6¾. State s Average shipping weight, 8 oz.

No. 40L710 Outfit, $2.85
Cadet Suit made of extra strong Galatea. Marine blue with silk braid trimming. Detachable brass buttons. Shoulder straps, slanting side pockets. Breast patch pockets with button flap. Straight style pants with white braid stripes at side. Side pockets. Cap, full lined, with sweatband. Imitation patent leather visor. Outfit consists of coat, pants and cap. SIZES—3 to 8 years. **State size.** Average shipping wt., 2¼ lbs.

No. 40L708 Outfit, $1.50
Military Play Suit made of olive drab cotton drill, trimmed with red. Military collar. Two side pockets. Brass buttons. Long pants have belt loops. Military stripe down side. Military full lined cap. Imitation patent leather visor. Brass emblems on cap and coat collar. Outfit consists of coat, pants and cap. SIZES—4 to 14 years. **State size.** Average shipping weight, 2¼ pounds.

No. 40L706 Outfit, $1.95
Military Outfit of khaki color strong cotton fabric. Military coat has four outside patch pockets with button flap. Pants with wide hips taper to lace below knee. Belt loops. Canvas leggings with strap for spiral wind. Cloth hat with stiff brim, full lined, sweatband. Haversack with shoulder strap. Outfit consists of coat, pants, hat, leggings and haversack. SIZES—5 to 11 years. **State size.** Av. shpg. wt., 2½ lbs.

No. 40L704 Outfit, $1.50
Rancher Cowboy Outfit. Strong khaki color cotton fabric. Shirt with breast pocket and imitation leather trimming. Long pants with belt loops. Imitation leather side trimmings with metal ornaments. Wide brim Western cloth hat, full lined. Outfit consists of shirt, pants, hat, red bandana handkerchief, belt with holster, toy pistol and roping lariat. SIZES—4 to 14 years. **State size.** Average shipping wt., 2¼ lbs.

No. 40L702 Outfit, $1.05
Pocahontas Indian Girl Suit. Blouse and skirt are made of khaki color cotton fabric. Navy blue V shape front, outlined with yellow and red trimmings. Sleeves trimmed in red. Eyelets for lacing front. Full cut skirt with red trimming at bottom. Headdress decorated with a number of large very highly colored feathers. SIZES—4 to 10 years. **State size.** Average shipping wt., 1½ lbs.

No. 40L700 Outfit, $1.05
Powhatan Big Chief Indian Outfit for boys. Made of olive khaki strong cotton drill. Scalloped red trimming. Navy blue V shaped front outlined with red and yellow trimming. Military eyelets for lacing. Long pants with belt loops. Warriors' headdress, trimmed from end to end with big brightly colored feathers. SIZES—4 to 10 years. **State size.** Average shipping weight, 1¼ pounds.

448 SEARS, ROEBUCK AND CO. CHICAGO. IMPORTANT! Be Sure to Read the Handy Post Cards Following Page 36

Courtesy Sears Graphics

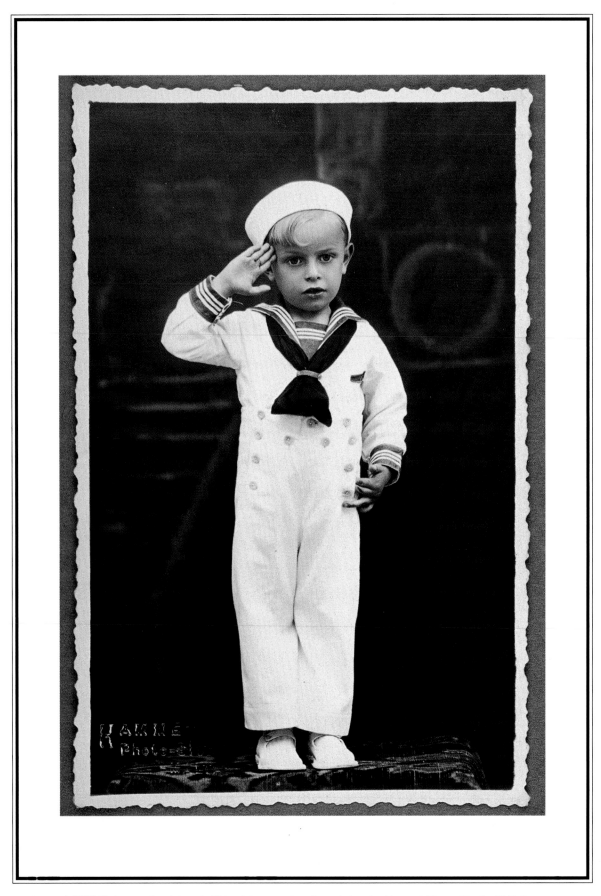

A WWI Maltese sailor (above). This picture postcard was taken by Hammt Photo Studio, Valletta, Malta. A small island nation in the Mediterranean, Malta was a British colony until 1961. An American boy (right) poses in a fashionable Navy-style suit with a flag in the background of this large-format (7" x 11½") patriotic image mounted on heavy mat board.

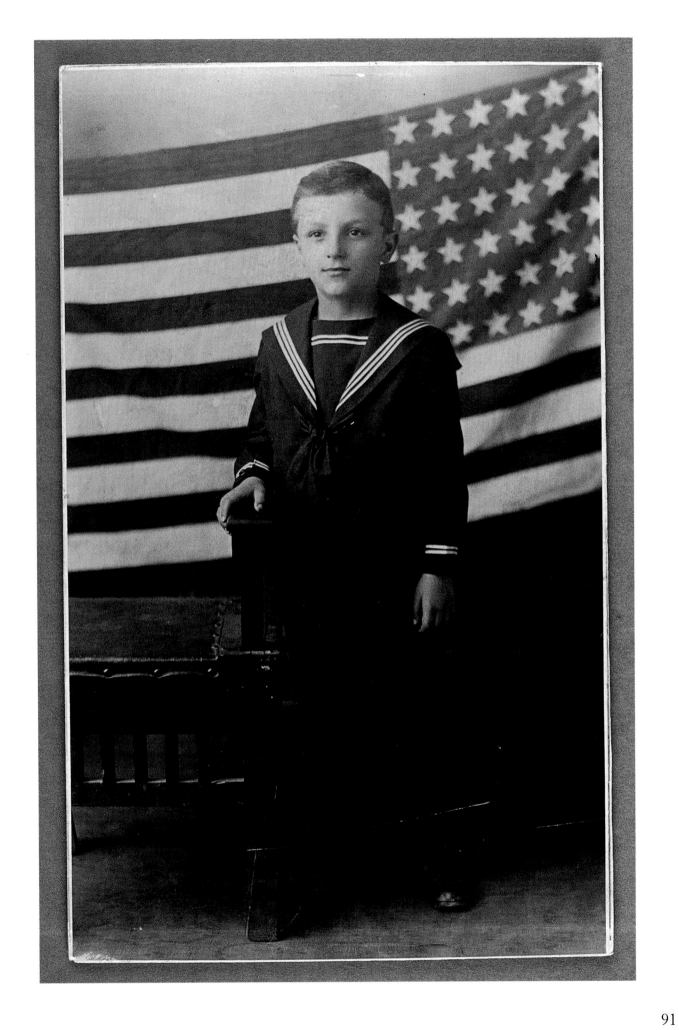

Whereas European children photographed in military-style costumes were generally children of significant means, as you will see later in this chapter, the heart of American patriotism becomes painfully evident when we observe this brave young soldier photographed in front of a dilapidated fence and unpainted house. The circumstances and elements of this photograph make it one of the most precious of the author's collection.

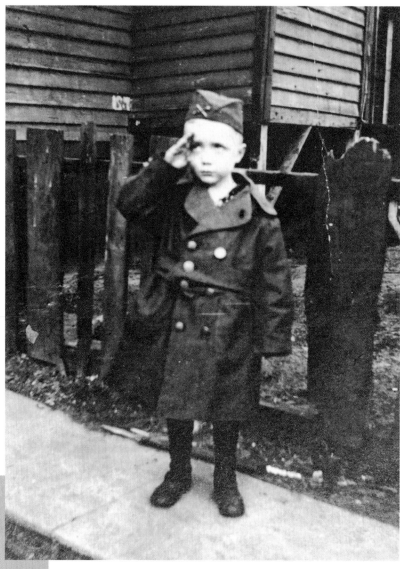

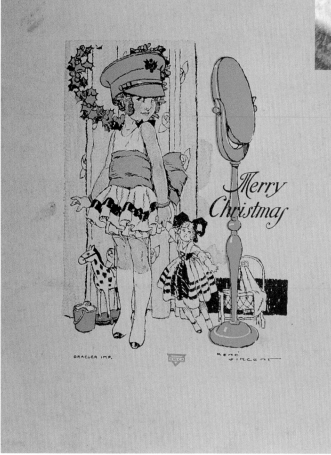

This postcard of a French girl in an American serviceman's hat is dated December 19, 1918, and was sent from "somewhere in France" to a child back in the States. Small cards such as this were provided by the YMCA and sent overseas to American soldiers who sent them home to friends and family at the holidays.

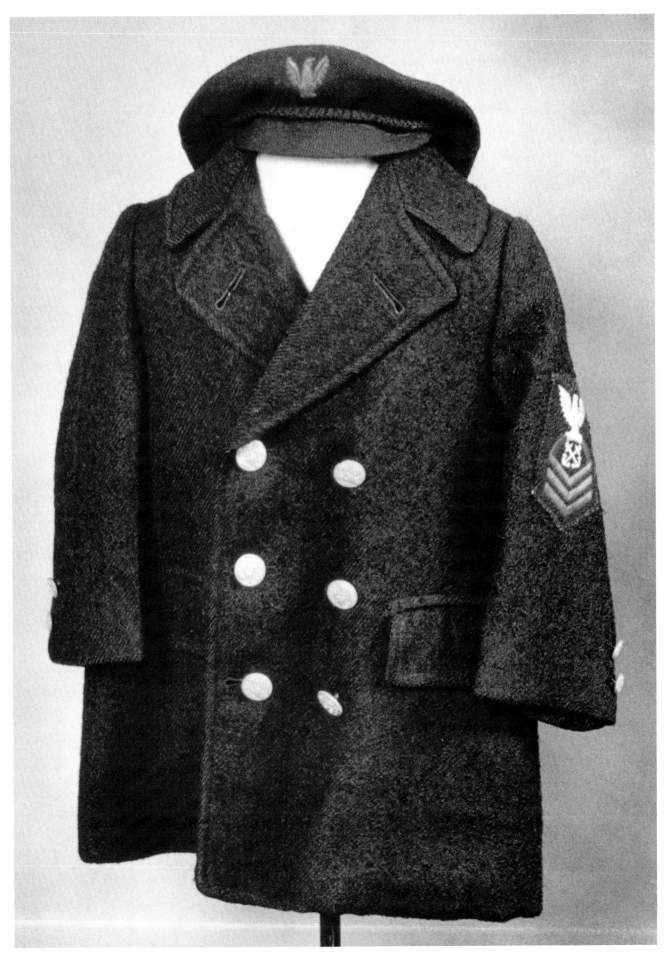

A cozy Navy pea coat and cap. The insignia on the sleeve is boatswain's mate or coxswain.

This series of commercial German postcards, circa WWI, depicts a boy mail carrier in a sailor-style blouse that carries a Reich's post bag.

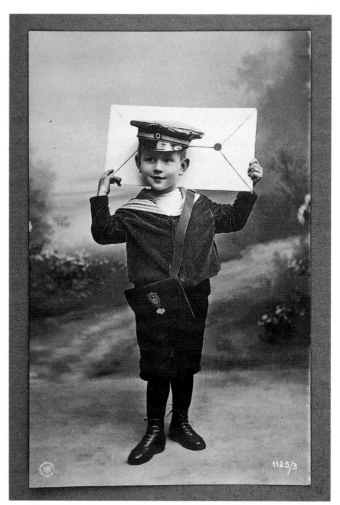

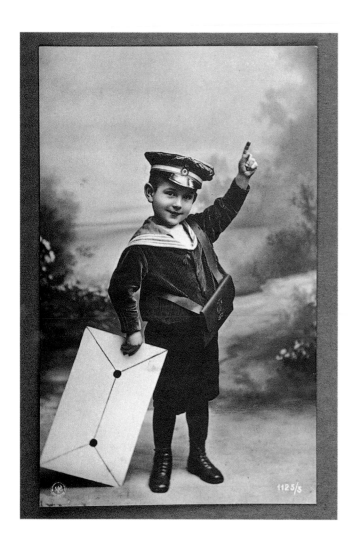

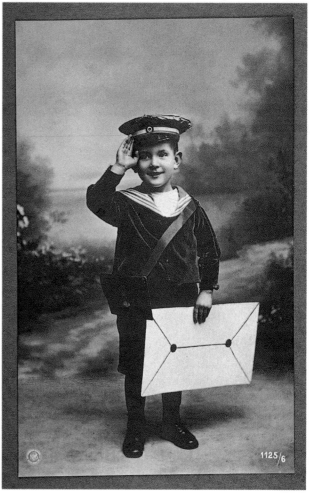

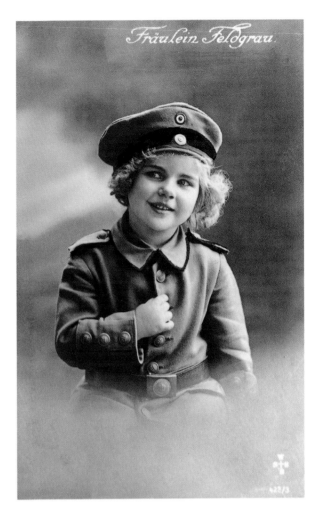

On the following pages are more commercially made German postcards, circa WWI. The children are dressed in remarkably accurate uniforms. They are well produced for the period, thus requiring little translation. The same models appear in a variety of military garb and different adult situations of wartime—from plotting where to make the strike, to the sentiments of missing a sweetheart, remembering the orphans, and complaining that the pay of a soldier allows for only one box of cigars a month.

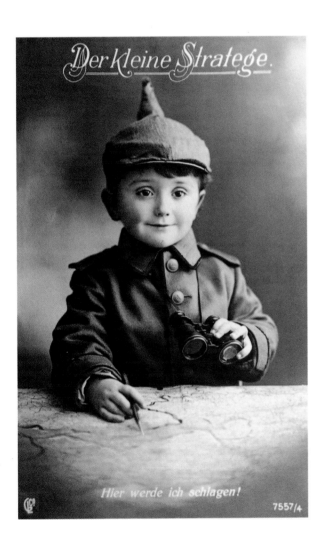

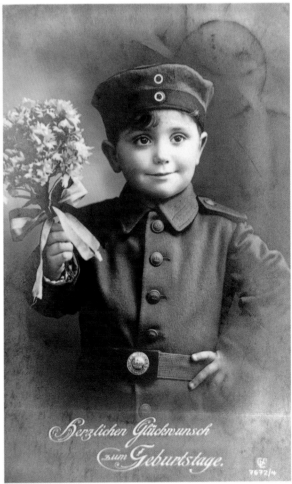

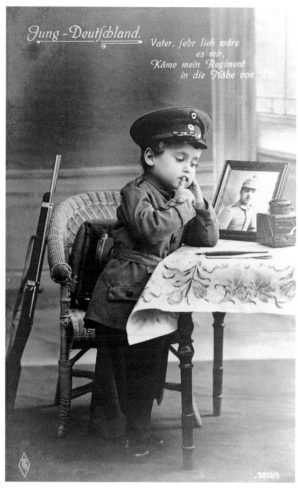

Jung-Deutſchland.

Vater, ſehr lieb wäre
es mir,
Käme mein Regiment
in die Nähe von Dir.

3872/5

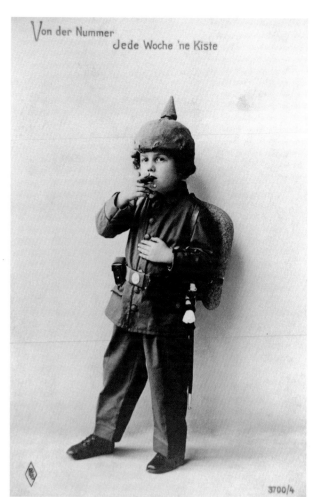

Von der Nummer
Jede Woche 'ne Kiste

3700/4

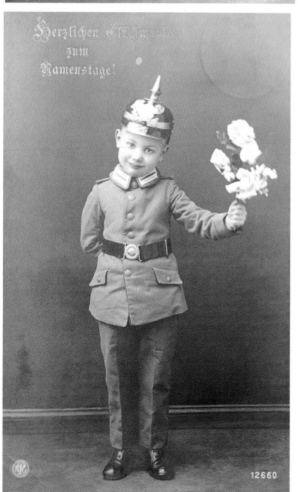

Herzlichen Glückwunſch
zum
Namenstage!

12660

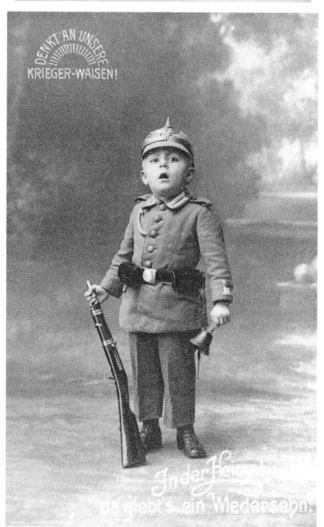

DENKT AN UNSERE
KRIEGER-WAISEN!

In der Heimat
da giebt's ein Wiederſehn

96

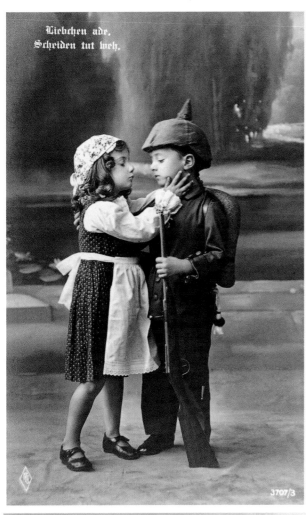

Liebchen ade.
Scheiden tut weh.

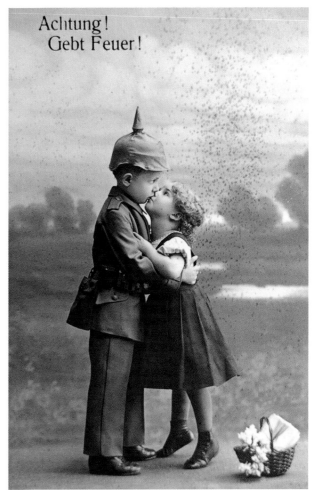

Achtung!
Gebt Feuer!

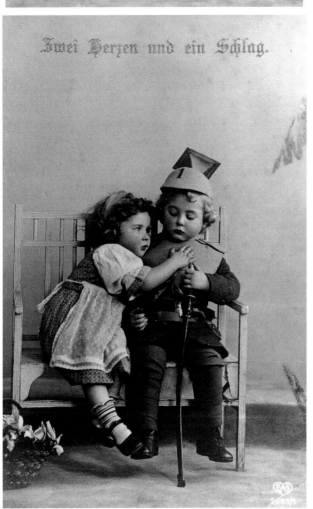

Zwei Herzen und ein Schlag.

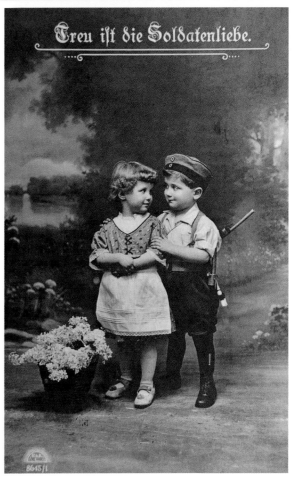

Treu ist die Soldatenliebe.

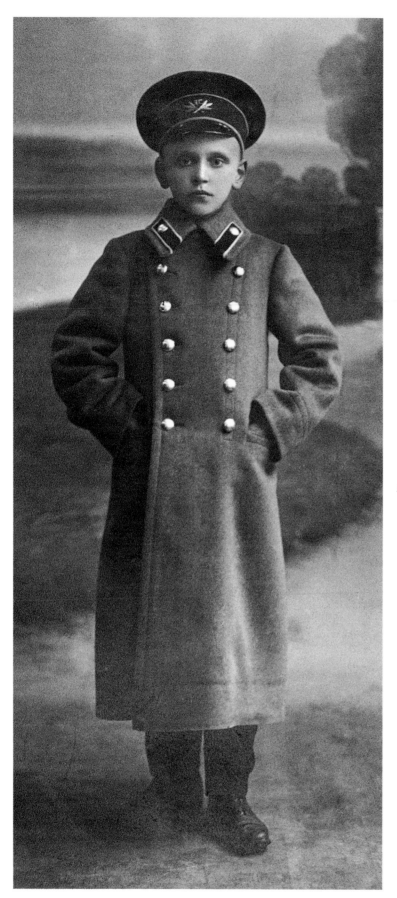

A boy WWI Russian military-style coat and hat in this Czechoslovakian picture postcard.

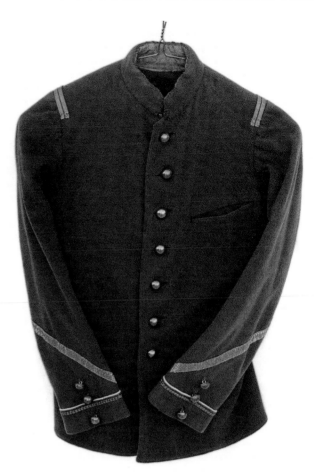

A French military-style tunic. *Courtesy Debra Allan Collection*

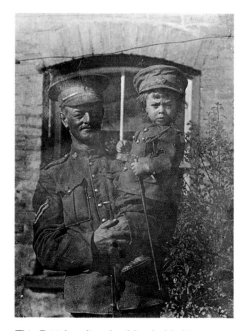

This British enlisted soldier holds his young son, who is dressed in an identical uniform.

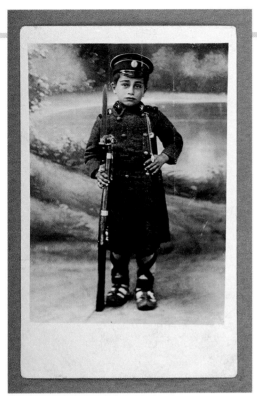

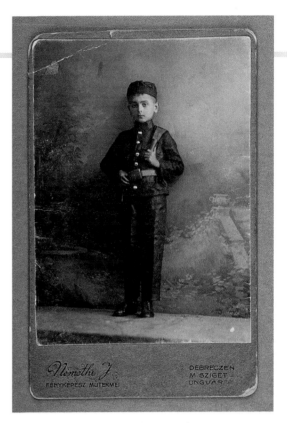

Another Russian boy in a picture postcard, with some portions hand-colored.

A Hungarian youth in a cabinet card image.

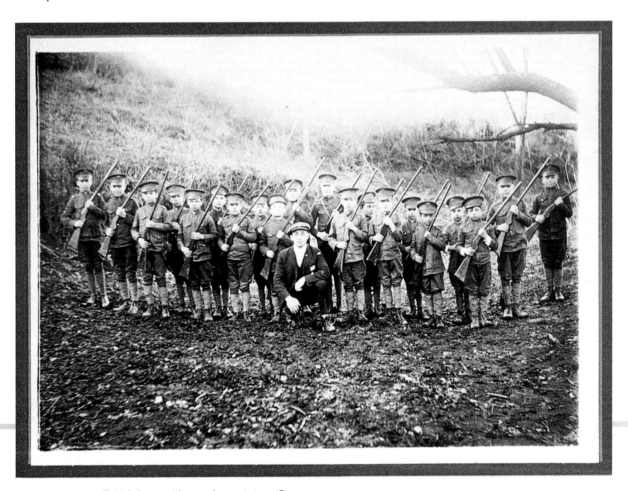

British boys with wooden training rifles.

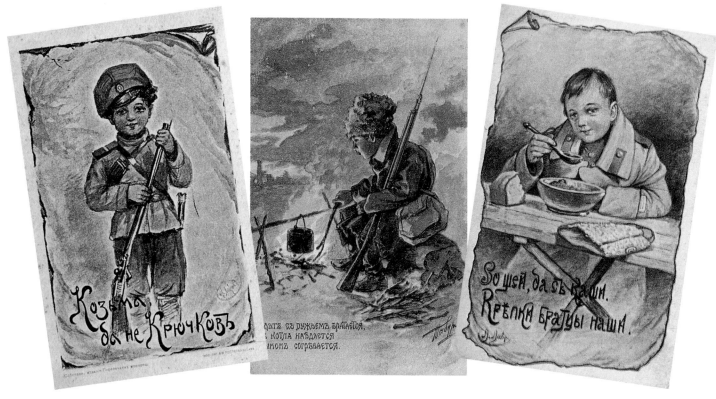

At left, "Kozma but not Kphkobt" (pronounced *kriptkoff*). Kozma Kphkobt is a Russian hero of the Imperial period who wielded a spear to kill offending German troops. At center, "The soldier fraternizes with his rifle, stuffs himself from the caldron and warms himself by the smoke" is by T. Kibble, artist; Petrograd (St. Petersburg) 50 Rubles for the benefit of the students." (Right) "With the soup and kasha [buckwheat] that's how our brothers pick up strength."

In this picture postcard dated April 24, 1917, a group of Russian soldiers pose with their regiment mascot in Kishinev, Moldavia (Chisinav). Note how the adult-size shoulder boards extend beyond the shoulders of this very young boy.

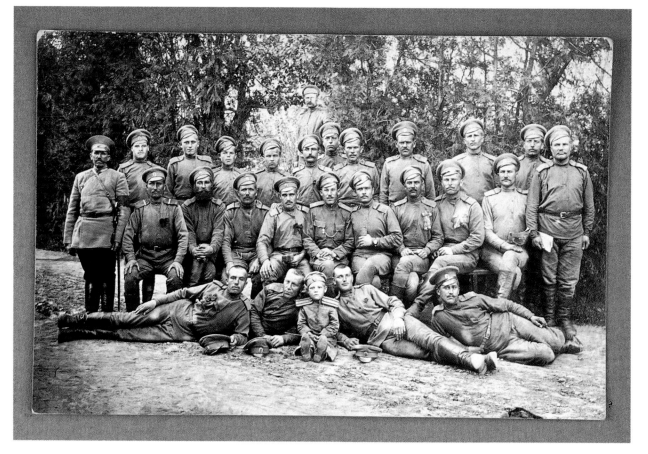

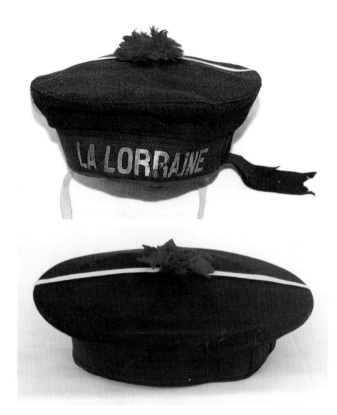

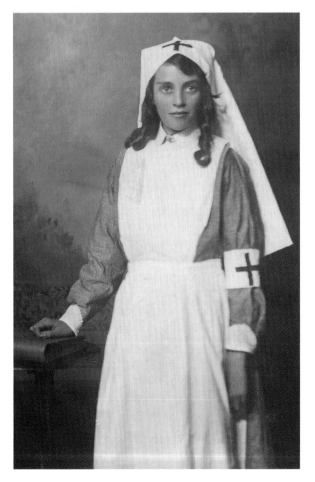

A pair of French Navy flat caps. As mentioned previously, in the 19th century, each French unit was attached to a particular city or port in the French republic.

It was popular for Australian girls to dress as nurses during WWI.

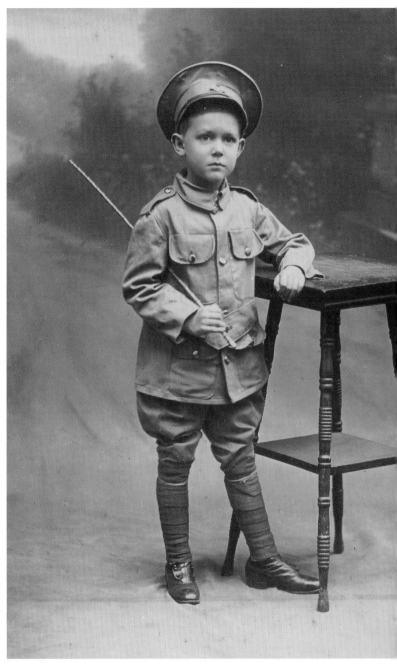

Enlisted Australian Army soldiers were referred to as "diggers." In WWI, the Army was called the 1st A.E.F. (Australian Expeditionary Forces). During World War II, it was called the 2nd A.E.F. This boy looks quite jaunty with his hat tipped slightly back and his swagger stick tucked deftly under his arm. *Courtesy Peter Coleman*

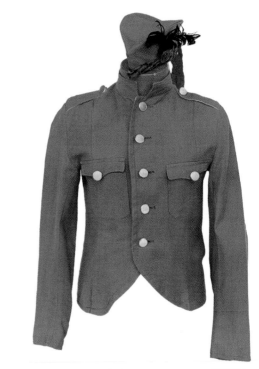

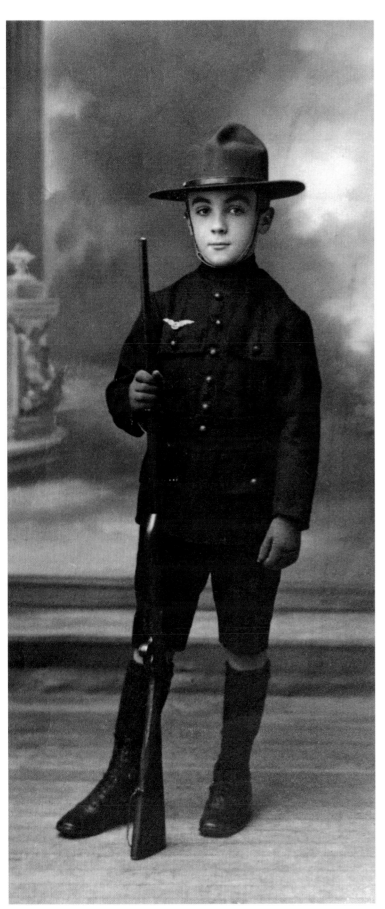

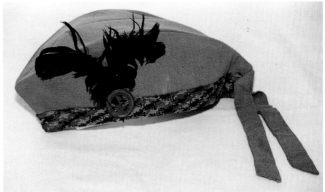

A Scottish uniform tunic and cap. The bottom of the tunic comes up in the center to accommodate the traditional kilt worn by soldiers. Elements of Scottish tradition such as the tartan band on the cap make this uniform very aristocratic. *Courtesy Debra Allan Collection*

WWI British tunic and visor cap. This outfit, which appears to be handmade, is of khaki cotton and is fully lined in cotton. The buttons appear to be replaced. It is sized to fit a boy of about eight or nine years old. *Courtesy Debra Allan Collection*

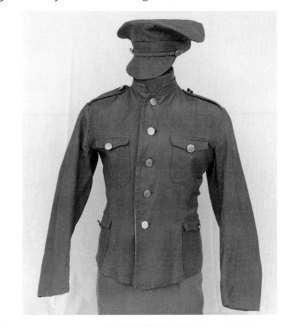

This French lad wears a WWI-style uniform with a wing of unknown origin. The back of the postcard reads, "Georges Morinet Gans, Hôtel Central, Orthez, B.F."

Four boys appear here dressed in a variety of French military-uniform styles from the WWI period. These trading cards were apparently a premium found in Maison Grondard Chocolate.

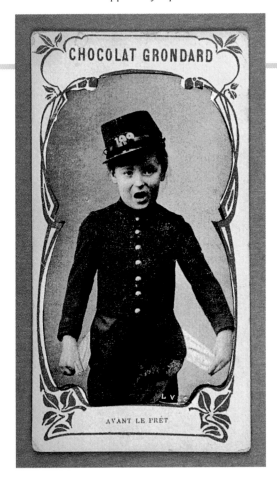

CHOCOLAT GRONDARD

AVANT LE PRÊT

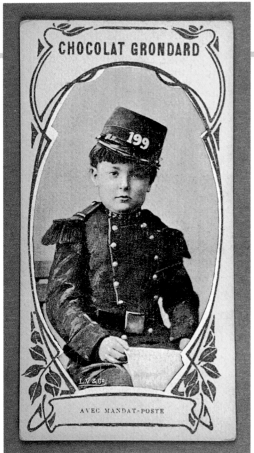

CHOCOLAT GRONDARD

AVEC MANDAT-POSTE

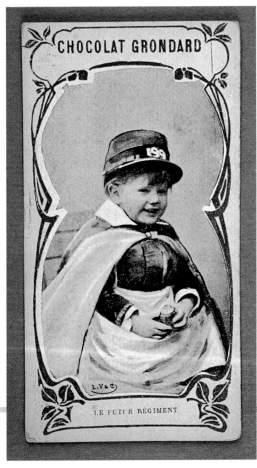

CHOCOLAT GRONDARD

LE FUTUR RÉGIMENT

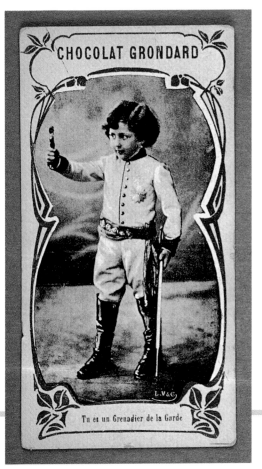

CHOCOLAT GRONDARD

Tu es un Grenadier de la Garde

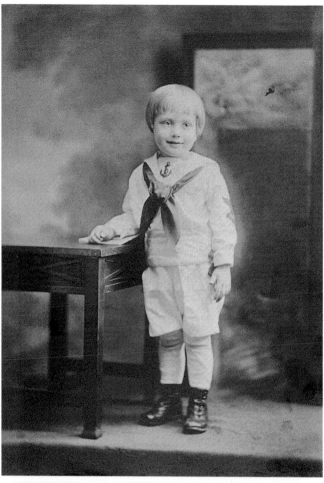

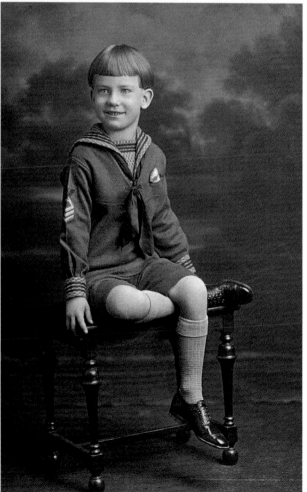

Unlike uniforms from Europe, American children's uniforms afforded a great deal of latitude in the way of interpretation. Textures, fabrics, and colors were rarely an issue when it came to a show of patriotism.

Left: Two happy sailors pose in studio setting photos.

Right: All the boys on this page have a common thread: a visor cap. Children of lesser means usually had to wear less expensive OS caps.

Note: the boy on the right in the lower left photo appears to be wearing an early interpretation of an aviator's uniform (see wings on the lapels). The buttons of his coat are set to one side, leaving room for a "map pocket" on the other. His little brother wears a terrifically oversized watch across his cuff.

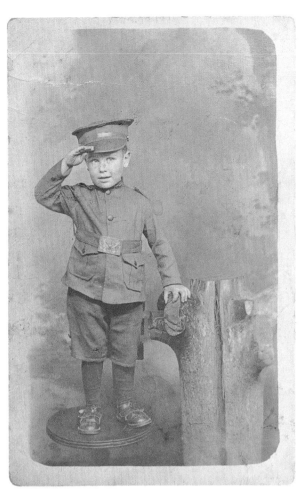

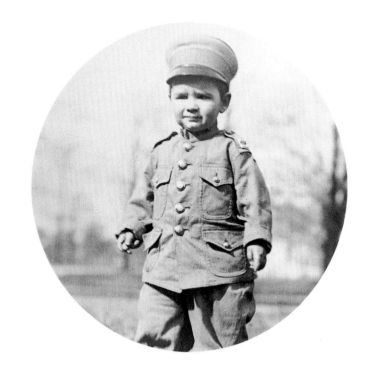

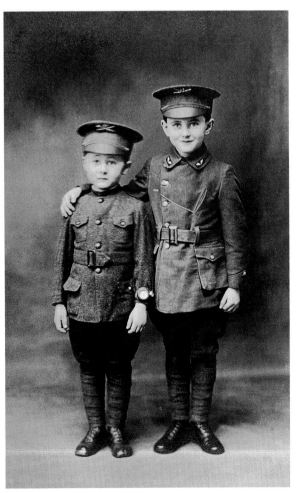

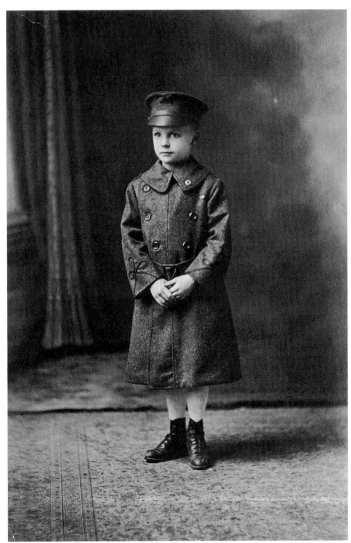

Between the Wars

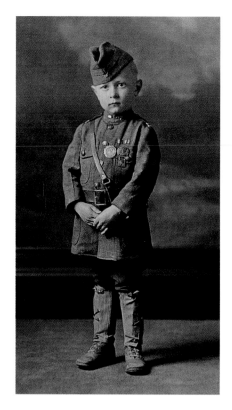

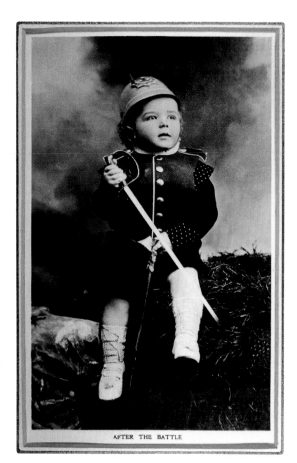

The back of this circa 1920 postcard reads, "To Uncle Dick and Aunt Norma from William Edward Boyer, age 3½ years. 100 percent Young America."

Another photo postcard, circa 1920, of a boy with a toy helmet, breastplate, and sword entitled "After the Battle." *Courtesy Michael J. Bremer*

AFTER THE BATTLE

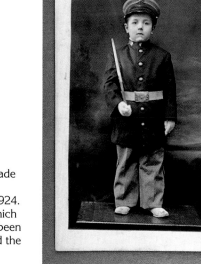

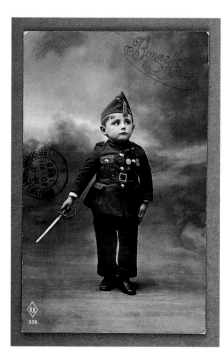

A terrific homemade outfit in a photo postcard dated 1924. Note the coat, which looks as if it has been pinned up around the hem.

An adorable hand-colored photo postcard from Brussels, Belgium, dated 1920. Note the incredibly short child's sword.

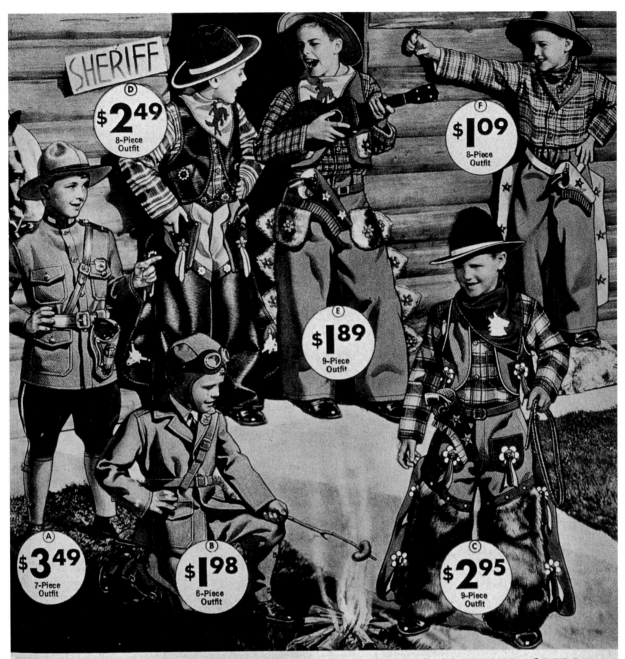

HOLIDAY ROUND-UP OF NOVELTY SUITS

(A) Monte the "Mountie"
• Coat of scarlet cotton twill with brass buttons—epaulets—and four pockets. "Mountie" insignia on collar and pocket. Navy blue cotton drill breeches. Brown cotton suede finish puttees. Large tan cotton suede cloth hat. Real leather Sam Browne belt and holster. Large toy pistol.
SIZES: 4, 6, 8, 10, 12, 14 yrs. *State age-size.* Shipping weight, 2 pounds 12 ounces.
40 V 4389—7-Pc. "Mountie" Outfit.............. **$3.49**

(D) Two-Gun Pete
• Brown imitation leather front chaps with two decorated holsters of cotton suede cloth. Plaid cotton flannel shirt • Imitation leather vest to match chaps • Gay Bandana • Two big "six-shooter" pistols • Lasso • Black cotton suede cloth hat.
Bang! Bang!—look out for Two-Gun Pete! He's got two big pistols to flourish!
SIZES: 4, 6, 8, 10, 12, 14 yrs. *State age-size.* Shipping weight, 3 pounds.
40 V 4375—8-Pc. Cowboy Outfit.............. **$2.49**

(B) The Flying Lieutenant
• Coat and breeches of tan khaki cotton drill • Two flap pockets • Flyer's insignia • Imitation leather Sam Browne belt and puttees • Helmet and goggles.
Young pilot's outfit! Trim fitting coat and breeches of sturdy khaki drill. Natty Sam Browne belt—and even a pair of goggles to shield your eyes from wind and glare.
SIZES: 4, 6, 8, 10, 12, 14 yrs. *State age-size.* Shipping weight, 2 pounds 12 ounces.
40 V 4353—6-Pc. Pilot's Outfit.. **$1.98**

(E) Dapper Dan
• Khaki cotton drill chaps with metal spangles—fur and leather trim. Bright plaid cotton flannel shirt.
• Fur decorated cotton khaki vest • Cotton khaki hat • Lasso. • Bandana.
• Large toy pistol and holster • Belt.
Dapper Dan wears a fur trimmed suit that's the envy of the whole corral! Vest has fur pockets—and chaps have fur side trimming.
SIZES: 4, 6, 8, 10, 12, 14 yrs. *State age-size.* Shipping weight, 2 pounds 12 ounces.
40 V 4366—9-Pc. Cowboy Suit. **$1.89**

(C) King of the Range
• Genuine fur front chaps • Plaid cotton flannel shirt • Large toy pistol and holster • Belt • Lasso • Black cotton suede cloth hat • Decorated khaki cotton drill vest • Colorful bandana.
Even your favorite cowboy movie star doesn't wear a finer outfit than this! The chaps are real fur. It's our finest suit.
SIZES: 4, 6, 8, 10, 12, 14 yrs. *State age-size.* Shipping weight, 3 lbs. 8 oz.
40 V 4370—9-Pc. Cowboy Outfit **$2.95**

(F) Broncho Bill
• Khaki cotton drill chaps with fancy side trim; elastic waist • Gay plaid cotton flannel shirt • Bright bandana.
• Cotton khaki cowboy hat • Belt, lasso, toy pistol, and holster.
Broncho Bill's outfit costs less, but it doesn't miss any of the trappings a cowboy should have. Chaps have fancy side decorations. Eight pieces included.
SIZES: 4, 6, 8, 10 yrs. *State age-size.* Shipping weight, 1 pound 12 ounces.
40 V 4363—8-Pc. Outfit...... **$1.09**

OTHER NOVELTY SUIT VALUES IN SEARS BIG CATALOG   SEARS ✓   PAGE **35**

Sears Christmas Wish Book 1937. *Courtesy Sears Graphics*

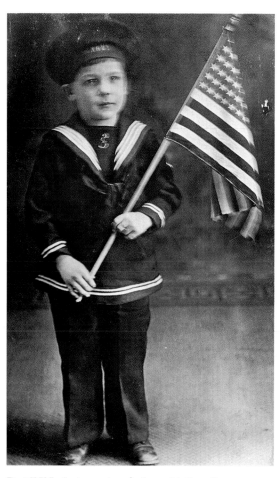

Post-WWI photo postcard of a patriotic sailor.

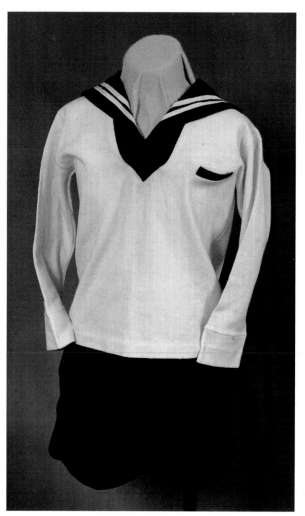

A lightweight wool Navy jumper and shorts, circa 1920s.

A beautiful studio portrait of brothers in linen/cotton sailor suits with plenty of detail.

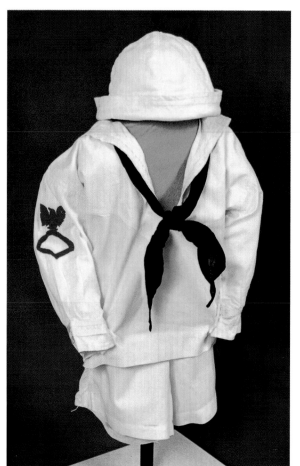

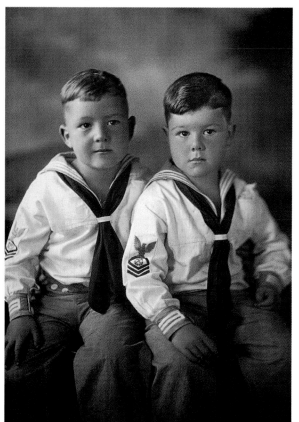

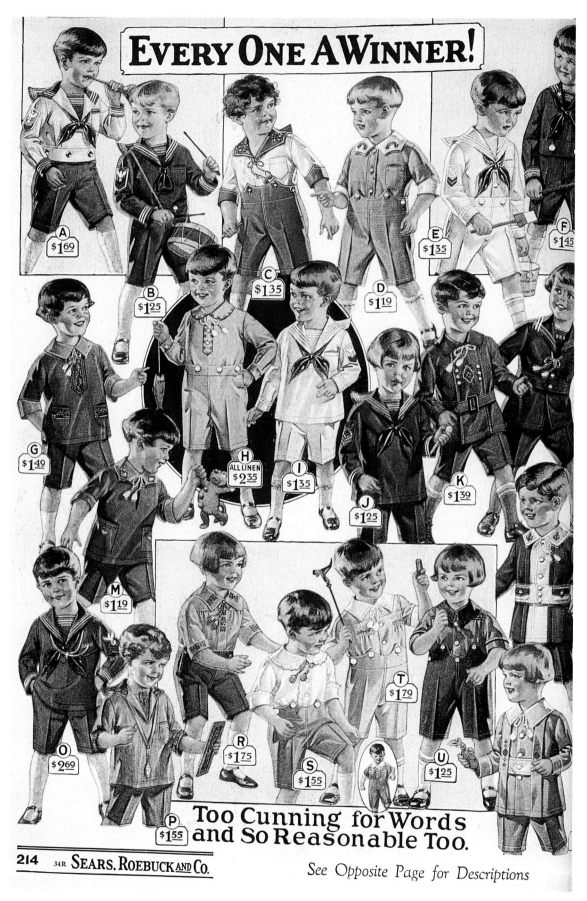

Too Cunning for Words and So Reasonable Too.

See Opposite Page for Descriptions

Collectors should not confuse fashion and suits or costumes made up to look like real uniforms. This page of children's sailor fashions is from the 1924 Spring Sears Roebuck Catalog. *Courtesy Sears Graphics*

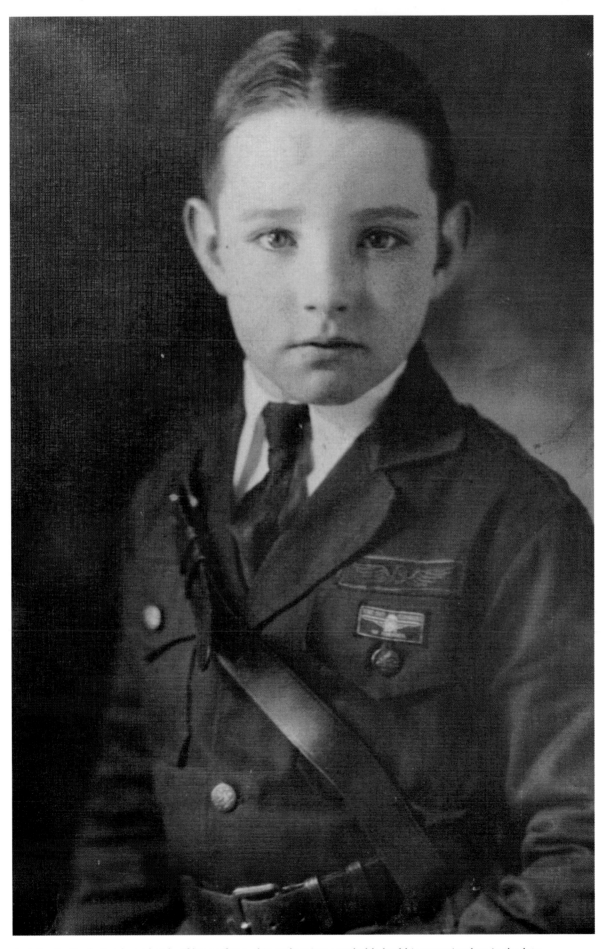

Judging by the hairstyle and style of his uniform, this early aviator probably had his portrait taken in the late 1920s when Lindbergh was all the rage. Note the two great fantasy patches on the breast of his coat.

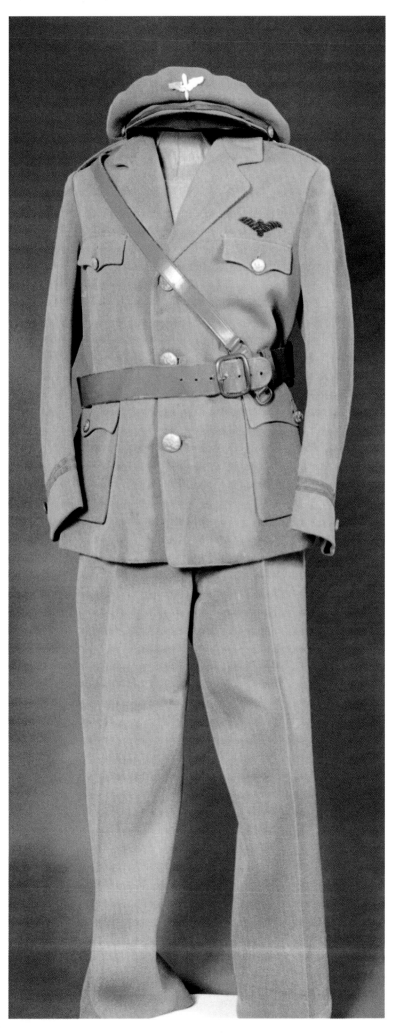

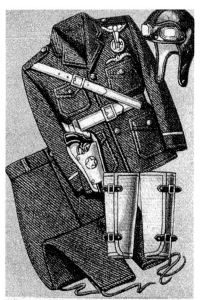

Montgomery Ward offered the
opportunity to "Be a Real Aviator" in
1940 with this uniform. *Courtesy
University of Wyoming American
Heritage Center*

Left:
This circa 1930s gabardine aviator's suit has been seen in
several fabric color variations of tan and green, with tailor
tags from New York to California. All have the distinctive
bullion wing and ribbon at the cuff stripes. The crusher cap
has an early Army Air Corps sweetheart winged propeller as
a cap emblem.

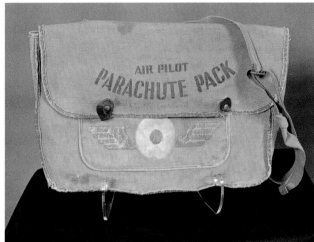

Air Pilot Parachute Pack, circa 1930s. Early winged roundel
insignia adds a classic touch for make-believe pursuit pilots.

A fabulous early aviator's suit. The many features include leather leggings, bullion wing, and military-style buttons, all of which make it very realistic. The disproportionately used gloves may have been added to the ensemble (period) to complete the effect. The overall style would suggest the early 1920s; however, the zippers on the trousers would date the suit in the 1930s when manufacturers first started using zippers on children's clothing. *Courtesy Rex Stark Americana*

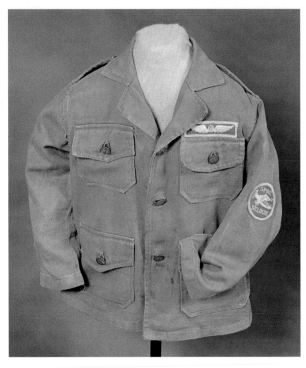

An olive-drab shirt celebrating aviation bears the same fantasy wing as the aviator portrait a few pages back. The *Spirit of St. Louis* patch dates from after 1927 when Charles Lindbergh made his historic transatlantic flight from New York to Le Bourget Field near Paris.

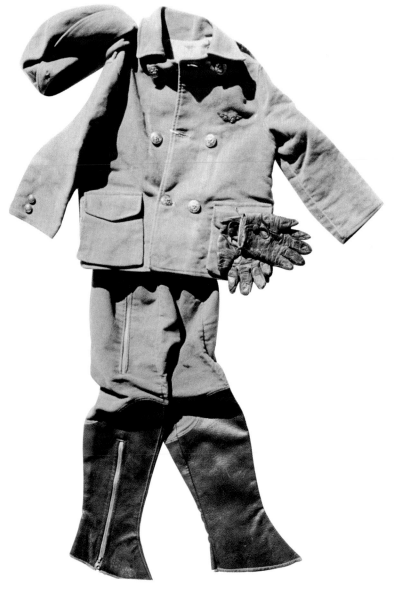

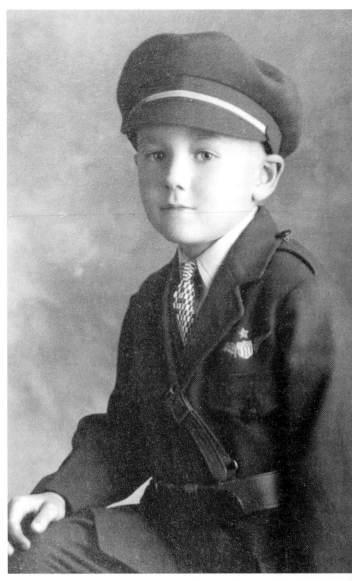

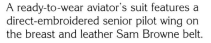

A ready-to-wear aviator's suit features a direct-embroidered senior pilot wing on the breast and leather Sam Browne belt.

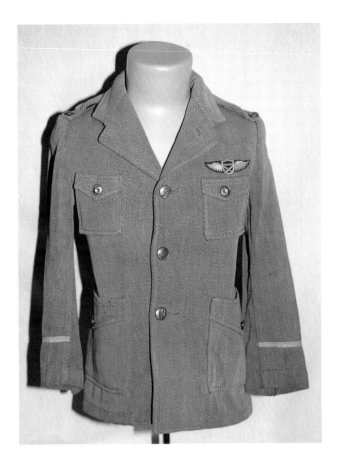

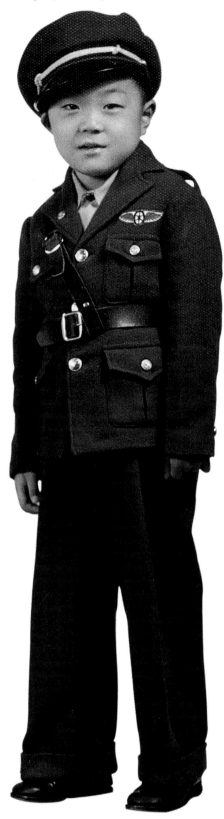

Though this photo (below) dates much later, the uniform is a style from the late 1930s to early 1940s. Perhaps it was handed down to a much younger brother or cousin? The two uniform coats (left) have some details such as cut, the wing style, and yellow cuff stripes. *Uniform top left courtesy Kathleen MacDonald Collection*

The maker label in this AAF tunic is Jackie Jumper, Registered, EE-Wald. *Courtesy Debra Allen Collection*

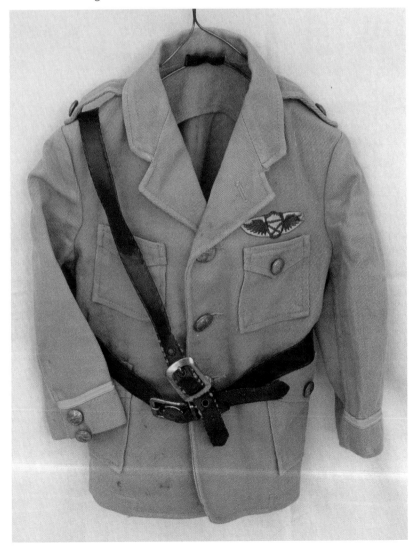

113

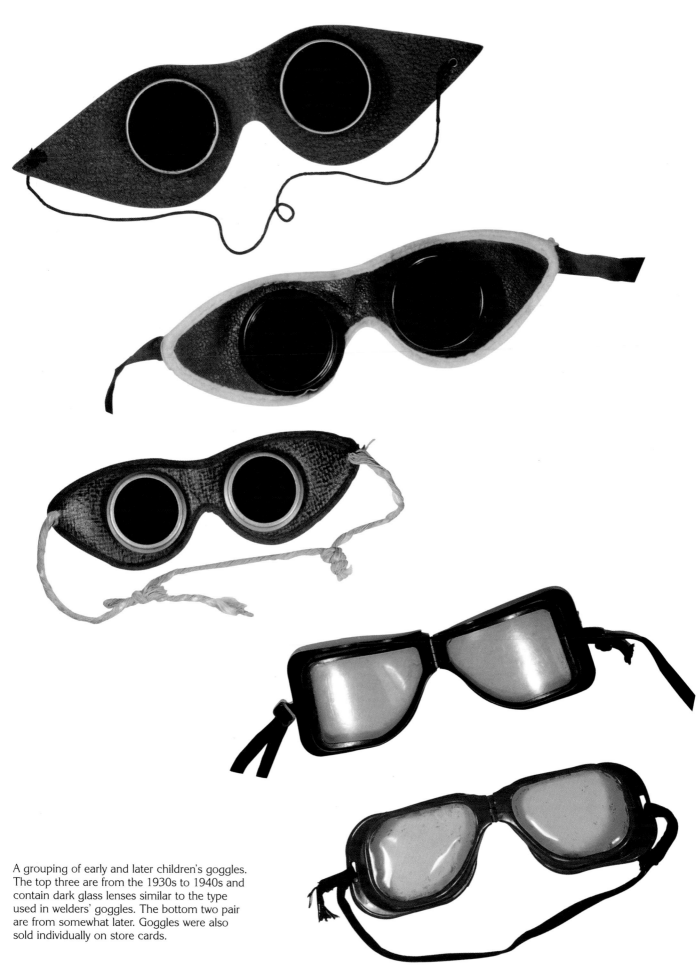

A grouping of early and later children's goggles. The top three are from the 1930s to 1940s and contain dark glass lenses similar to the type used in welders' goggles. The bottom two pair are from somewhat later. Goggles were also sold individually on store cards.

114

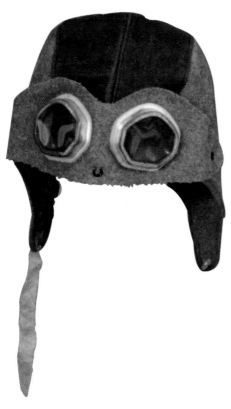

A woolen felt flying helmet with attached goggles.

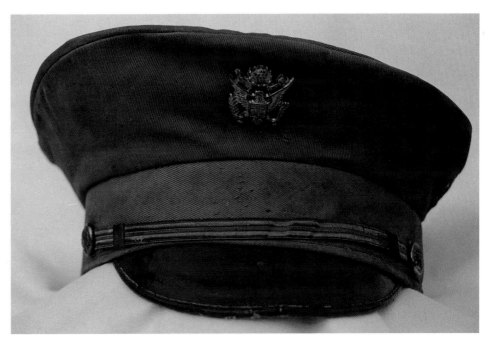

Army leather visor cap in wanting condition with insignia, military-style buttons, and gold bullion ribbon on the brim. This is probably the lone surviving piece left from a uniform ensemble.

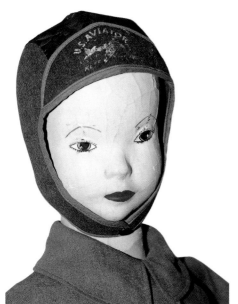

A terrific two-tone wool felt child's aviator helmet with button closure. *Courtesy Kathleen MacDonald Collection*

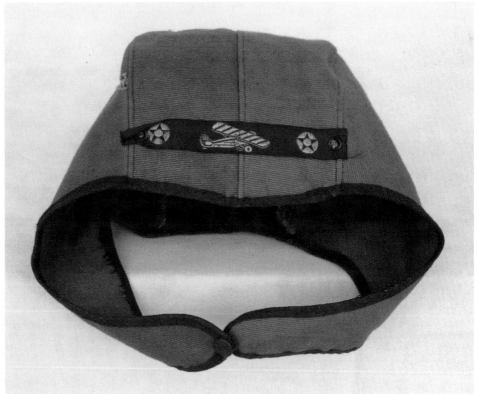

An early olive-drab twill aviator's cap is decorated with a ribbon and button closure. *Courtesy Debra Allen Collection*

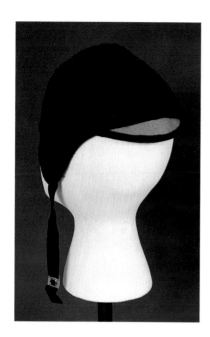

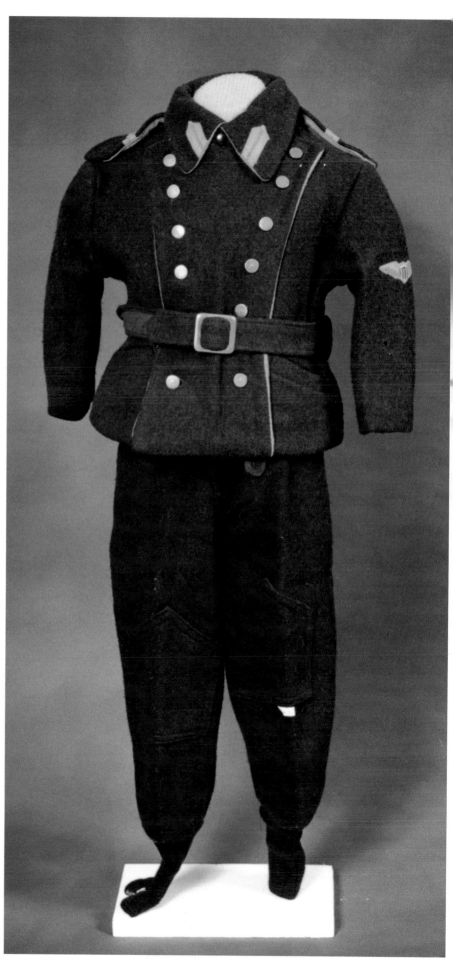

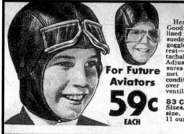

Snow hats are aviators' helmets in the eyes of a boy in 1937. *Courtesy Sears Graphics*

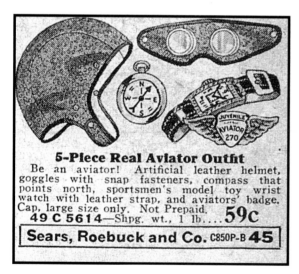

Circa 1936. *Courtesy Sears Graphics*

Someone added ribbons to the collar and epaulettes, and a fantasy wing to the sleeve of this thick woolen snowsuit. The helmet-style aviator cap (left) completes the look.

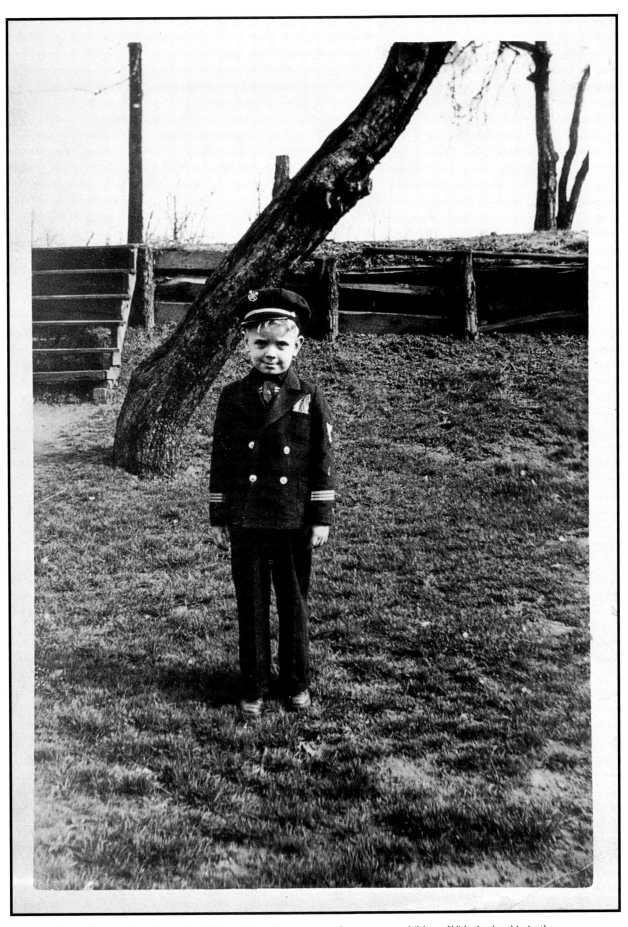

This handsome Navy-style suit is quite different from those most often seen on children. With the hankie in the breast pocket, it nearly resembles a yachting outfit. Note the coxswain emblem on the visor cap.

Part Two: 1941-1976
An Introduction⸺

Jack Matthews

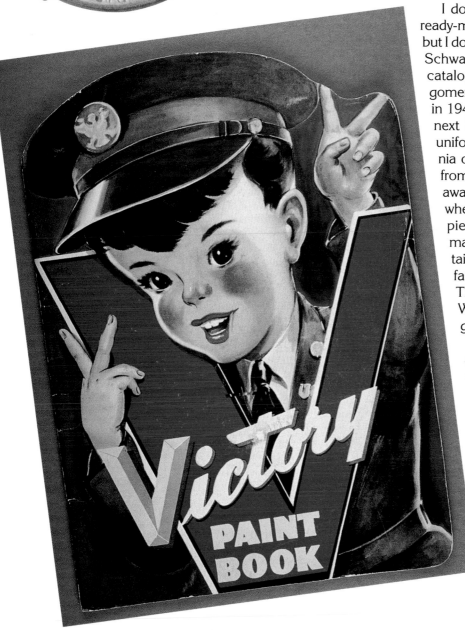

Once upon a very long time ago, way back during World War II, I played soldier all day long. I was nine years old. Within months after the dastardly sneak attack by the Japanese on Pearl Harbor, my chums and I went on "active duty" in our small New England town. Trenches and foxholes were dug in. Backyard observation posts were built in apple trees, and Boy Scout pup-tent bivouacs set up. Since we were growing boys, emergency rations of saltines, peanuts, raisins, and cookies were hidden under front steps and back porches.

I don't recall if my platoon ever wore ready-made manufactured kid's uniforms, but I doubt it. We had never heard of F.A.O. Schwarz, but the Christmas Wishbook catalogs of Sears Roebuck and Montgomery Ward did start showing uniforms in 1942. Instead, my gang and I did the next best thing. We created our own uniforms. Fascinated by military insignia of all kinds, we fashioned our own from examples in numerous free, give-away pamphlets available almost anywhere. With a box of crayons and a piece of cardboard, it was easy to make private-first-class stripes, captains' bars, and the like, and pin or fasten them on with rubber bands. Throw in a small-size surplus World War I helmet, and you had the beginnings of a uniform!

One of the most fascinating aspects of World War II is how children adapted to that horrible episode in our history. Engaging in a fantasy land of war play was a logical escape, and many boys did just that. For children of this era, being bathed in the patriotic spirit was almost a daily occurrence. Imagine, if you will, children in their makeshift uniforms stopping to reverently salute soldiers walking down the street or pushing to the front of a crowded train station and waving flags to greet a train of homecoming heroes. It is a time in our history the likes of which we will probably never see again.

What you will find in Part Two of this book is both a compelling and fascinating visual history of uniforms and toys from the years 1941 to 1976. The breadth and depth of Nancy's and her contributors' collections is stunning. Particularly appealing are the hundreds of photos of the kids themselves grandly arrayed in their uniforms. See the proud looks on their faces, and imagine their delight, to say nothing of the delight of beaming parents behind the camera lenses. The number and variety of photos and uniforms of children from all World War II countries—friend and foe—are astounding. If you are like me, you'll immediately want to frame half the images.

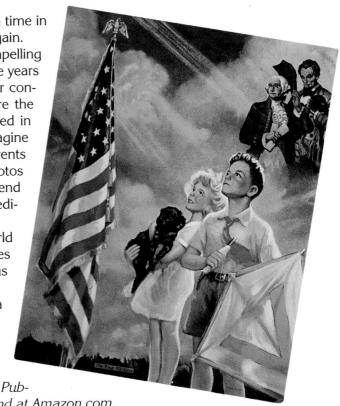

For a man who has collected well over a thousand World War II toys over the years and who is still finding treasures through the miracle of the Internet, this book is a marvelous surprise.

I thought I knew a lot about this stuff, but now I know a lot, lot more!

Jack Matthews is the author of the best-selling full-color book on World War II toys, puzzles, games, and children's books Toys Go To War, 1944, *Pictorial Histories Publishing Company, Missoula, Montana, which can be found at Amazon.com.*

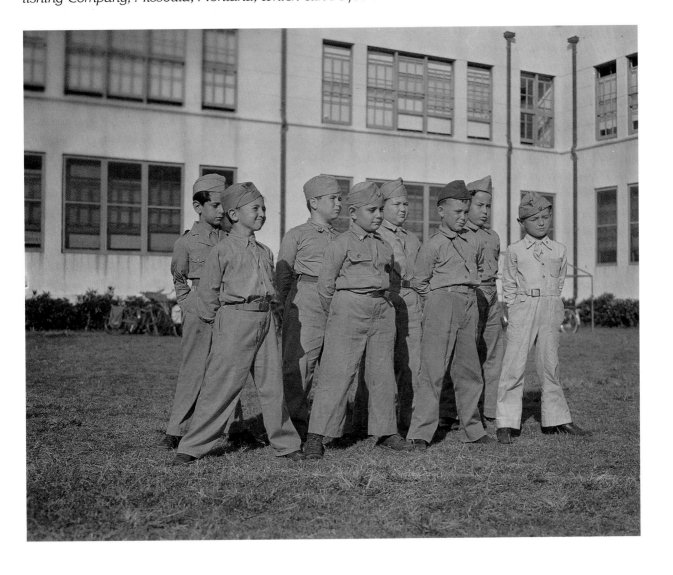

Chapter 8

1941-1945 V...

A pair of 3rd Air Force uniforms in brown wool tweed. When we compare the two, vast differences in accessories are evident. Manufacturers substituted whatever was on hand when appointed accessories ran out. You may see Navy-style buttons or insignia on Army uniform styles. In this case, military-style buttons appear on the example at left but not on the example on the right. Fabrics may vary and other accoutrements (insignia, belts, hats, etc.) may or may not be included, even when mint-in-the-box examples are found. *Example left courtesy Kathleen MacDonald Collection*

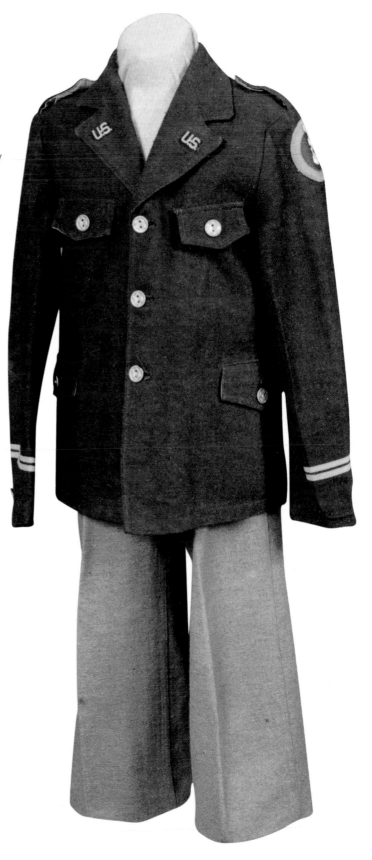

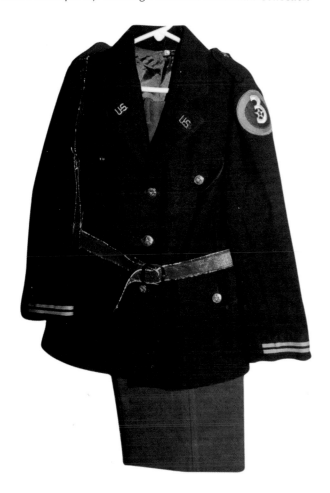

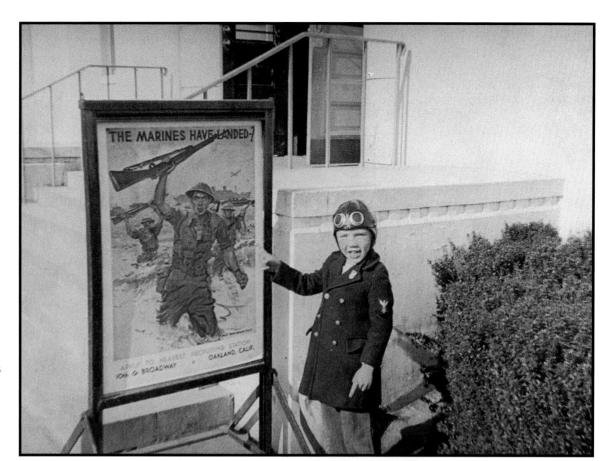

In this hand-colored photograph, a boy in front of a WWII Oakland, California, recruiting station poses in his Navy pea coat and aviator's helmet.

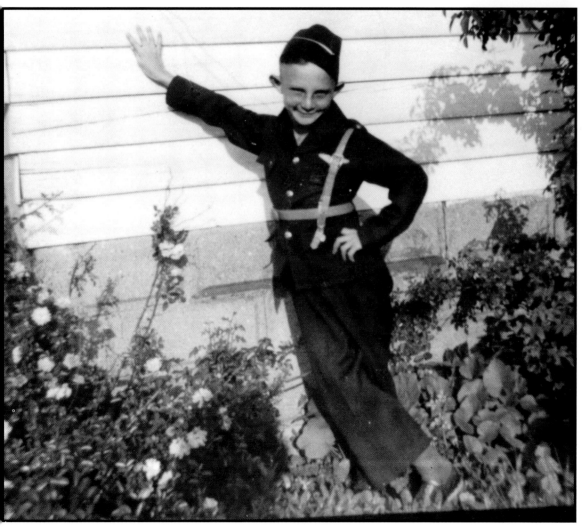

Wearing his Sam Browne belt on the wrong side (notice how it covers his wing) doesn't seem to bother the nine-year-old boy in this circa 1942 image. *Courtesy Kathleen MacDonald Collection*

121

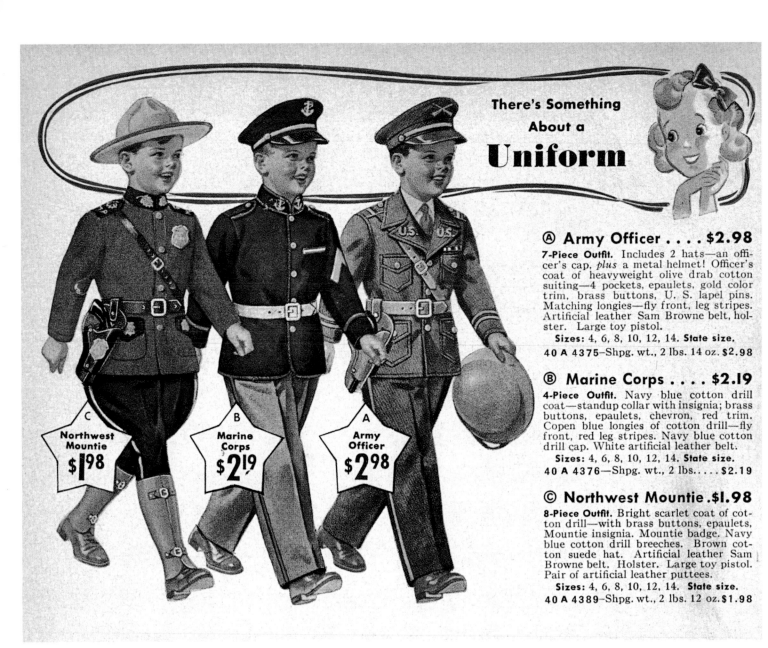

There's Something About a **Uniform**

Ⓐ Army Officer $2.98

7-Piece Outfit. Includes 2 hats—an officer's cap, *plus* a metal helmet! Officer's coat of heavyweight olive drab cotton suiting—4 pockets, epaulets, gold color trim, brass buttons, U. S. lapel pins. Matching longies—fly front, leg stripes. Artificial leather Sam Browne belt, holster. Large toy pistol.

Sizes: 4, 6, 8, 10, 12, 14. **State size.**
40 A 4375–Shpg. wt., 2 lbs. 14 oz. $2.98

Ⓑ Marine Corps $2.19

4-Piece Outfit. Navy blue cotton drill coat—standup collar with insignia; brass buttons, epaulets, chevron, red trim. Copen blue longies of cotton drill—fly front, red leg stripes. Navy blue cotton drill cap. White artificial leather belt.

Sizes: 4, 6, 8, 10, 12, 14. **State size.**
40 A 4376–Shpg. wt., 2 lbs. $2.19

Ⓒ Northwest Mountie . $1.98

8-Piece Outfit. Bright scarlet coat of cotton drill—with brass buttons, epaulets, Mountie insignia. Mountie badge. Navy blue cotton drill breeches. Brown cotton suede hat. Artificial leather Sam Browne belt. Holster. Large toy pistol. Pair of artificial leather puttees.

Sizes: 4, 6, 8, 10, 12, 14. **State size.**
40 A 4389–Shpg. wt., 2 lbs. 12 oz. $1.98

C Northwest Mountie $1.98

B Marine Corps $2.19

A Army Officer $2.98

Circa 1941. With an escalating war in Europe, national interest turns to defense. Sears, Roebuck & Co. returns the play uniforms, not seen since 1938, to the Christmas Wish Book . *Courtesy Sears Graphics*

Circa 1942. 1941 Congressional Acts "L" (limitation) and "M" (conservation) limited toy manufacturer's use of raw materials. Reduced by one piece, the Army Officer's uniform set is absent the metal doughboy helmet offered in the same ensemble a year earlier. (Left) Toy manufacturers were allowed to use raw materials appearing on the prohibited list until June 30, 1942 and were not required to turn in completed toys for conversion to other uses. Sales of completed metal toys lasted only a few months, giving way to new toys manufactured from "nonessential" materials such as wood, plastic, and cardboard for the duration of the war. Courtesy Sears Photo Archives.

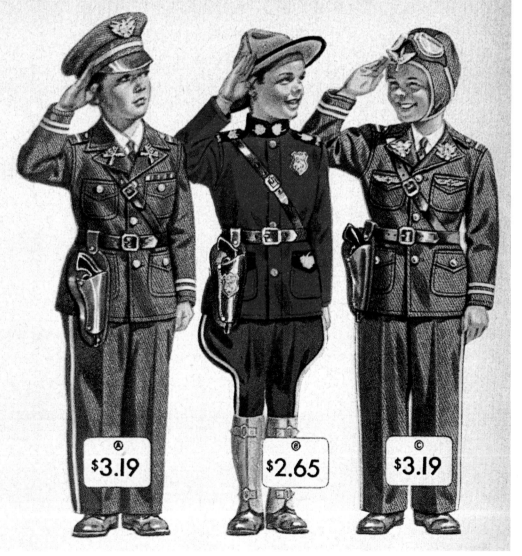

Snappy Uniforms FOR YOUNG AMERICANS

Army Officer . . . 6 pieces

(*A*) Heavy olive drab cotton twill. Coat **$3.19** with 4 pockets; epaulets; gold color braid, buttons, and crossed rifle lapel pins. Fly front longies. Matching officer's cap with insignia. Artificial leather Sam Browne belt, holster. Toy pistol. *State size.*
   Even sizes only: 4 to 14.
40 P 4360—Wt., 2 lbs. 14 oz.

Northwest Mountie . . . 8 pcs.

(*B*) Sturdy cotton drill, Scarlet coat **$2.65** with brass color buttons, epaulets, Mountie insignia. Mountie badge. Navy blue breeches. Brown cotton suede hat. Artificial leather Sam Browne belt, holster, and pair puttees. Toy pistol. *State size.*
   Even sizes only: 4 to 14.
40 P 4389—Wt., 2 lbs. 12 oz.

Flying Cadet . . . 7 pieces

(*C*) Strong olive drab cotton drill. Coat **$3.19** has 4 pockets; epaulets; gold color trim. Fly front longies, braid leg stripes. Matching aviators helmet with insignia. Goggles. Artificial leather Sam Browne belt, holster. Large toy pistol. *State size.*
   Even sizes only: 4 to 14.
40 P 4358—Wt., 2 lbs. 14 oz.

Ⓐ $3.19   Ⓑ $2.65   Ⓒ $3.19

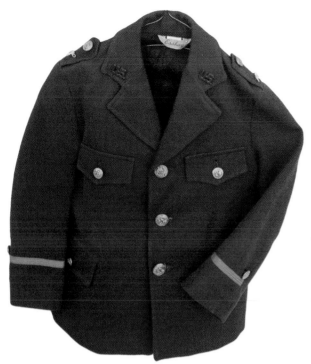

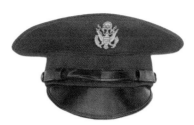

Army tunic and cap. The brown twill tunic has military-style buttons, U.S. collar insignia, and eagle devices on the epaulettes. The label inside the collar reads: "Esskay, Size 3, lot 4856." The visor cap is brown twill with leatherette chin strap and visor. It is maker marked "Goldsmith's-Memphis Greatest Store, size 6½." *Courtesy Debra Allan Collection*

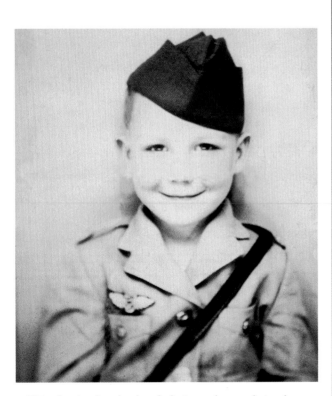

This pleasing hand-colored photograph was obviously carried in a wallet for a very long time.

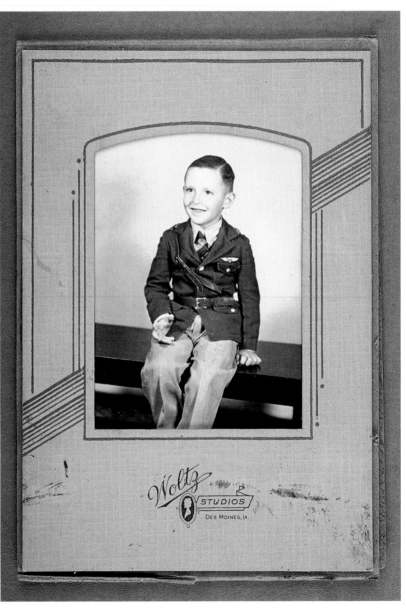

A young aviator, with slicked hair and "non-regulation" shirt and tie, smiles for the camera at Woltz Studios in Des Moines, Iowa.b

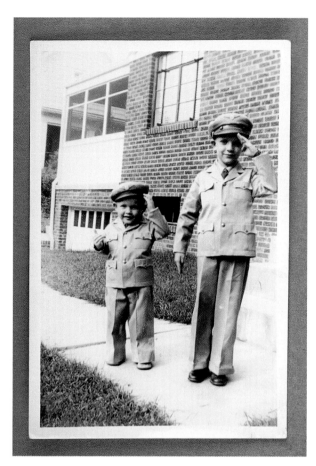

These saluting brothers in matching aviator suits were snapped in front of their home in August 1942.

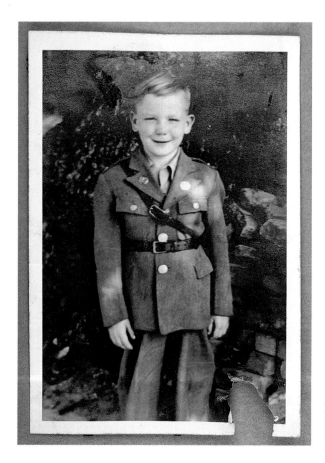

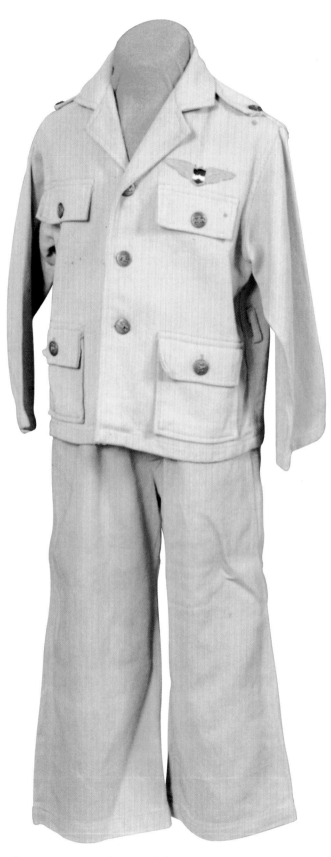

A tan cotton aviator's suit with fantasy wing insignia.

Paul Barrett of Chicago, Illinois, was photographed in 1945 in his fine Army uniform adorned with genuine enlisted-man's collar insignia. *Courtesy Mike Constable*

A commercial khaki Air Force tunic, trousers, and leatherette visor cap with insignia. Note that someone has added an Army/Air Force shoulder patch to this well-made ensemble.

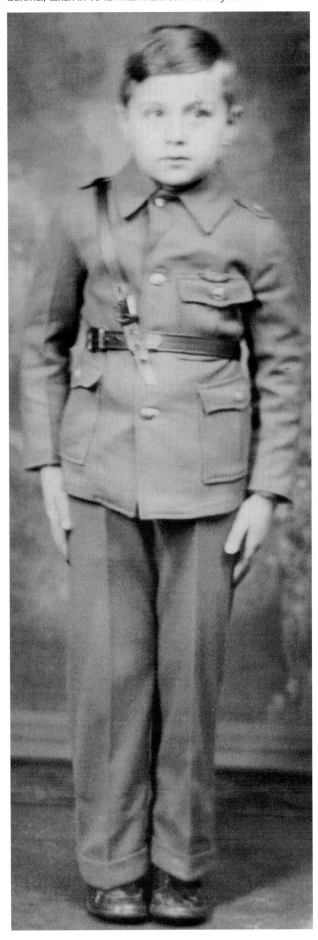

Caryl Young contributed this photograph of her cousin, Kenneth Sohmer, taken in 1942 when Kenneth was six years old.

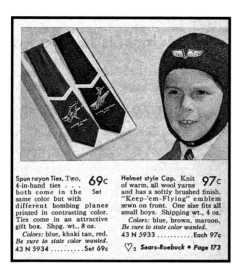

Courtesy Sear Graphics

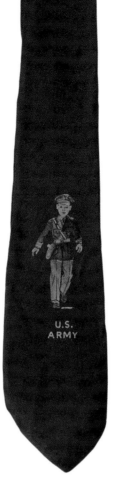

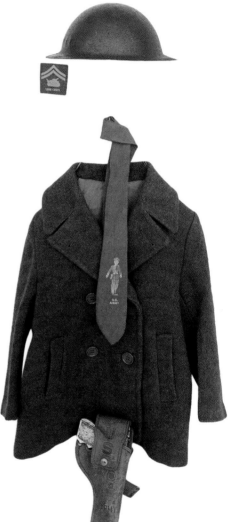

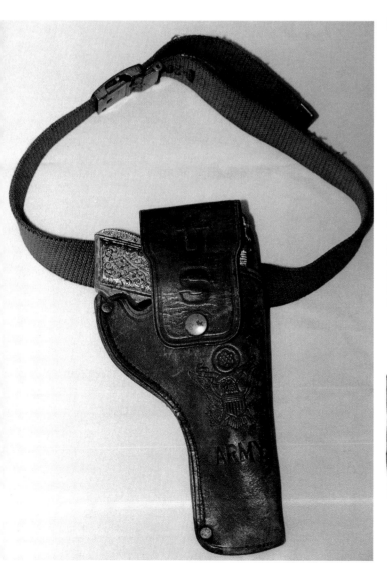

A terrific Army grouping from the collection of Debra Allan, including an olive-drab overcoat identical to an adult version, red "Army" tie, officer's .45 with holster, and fantasy tanker's patch.

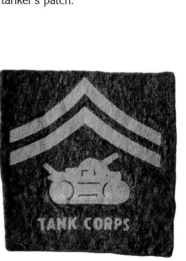

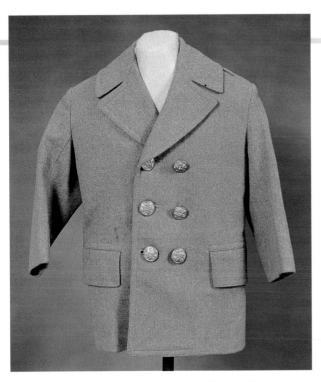

Another OD wool Army overcoat with military-style buttons. At one time it bore a shoulder patch that has since been removed.

A home-grown green wool U.S.M.C. outfit complete with shirt-size EGAs (Eagle, Globe, and Anchor) added to the lapels and helmet. *Courtesy Debra Allan Collection*

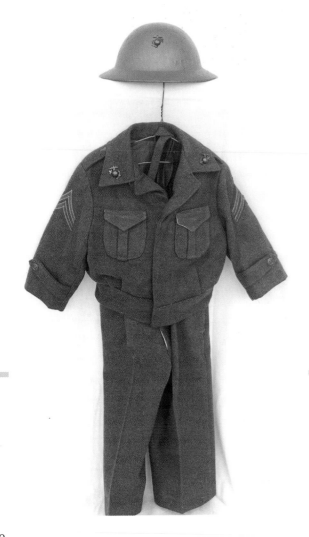

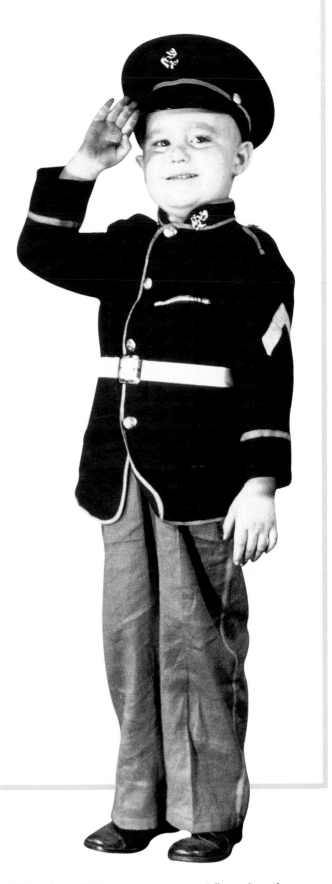

This saluting Marine wears a commercially made uniform with play EGA devices on the visor cap and collars.

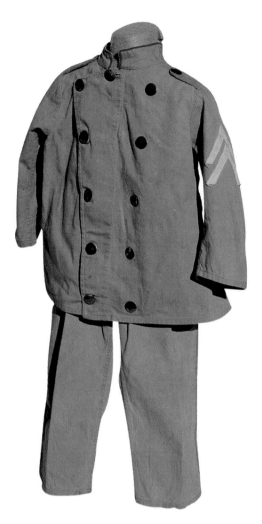

Highly stylized khaki-colored uniform with sleeve insignia and doubled-breasted front.

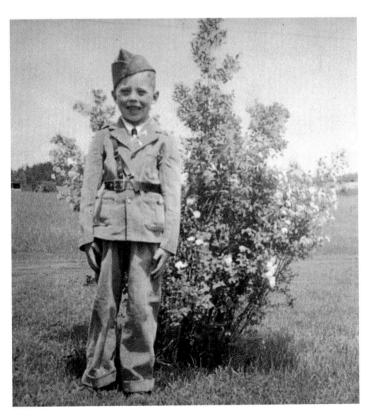

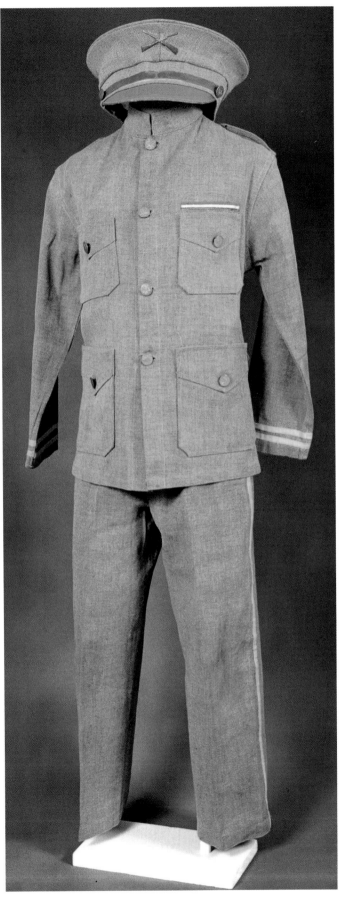

An early WWII-style brown wool-blend uniform with stamped, military-style buttons. The crossed rifles have either been added or crudely reattached to the hat.

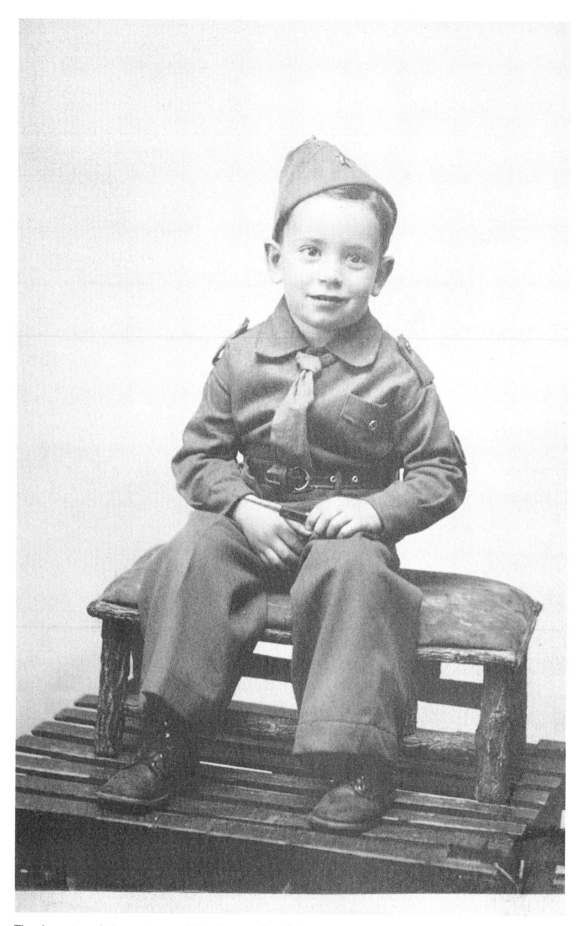

The elements and circumstances of this photograph make it very curious to the author. The Army-style uniform appears to be a conglomeration of store-bought and homemade pieces for just the right effect. But the shoes are obviously very worn, and the pedestal and bench are quite shabby, making one wonder what the economic status of this Pennsylvania boy was in 1944. *Courtesy Cocoa Curio, Hershey, Pennsylvania*

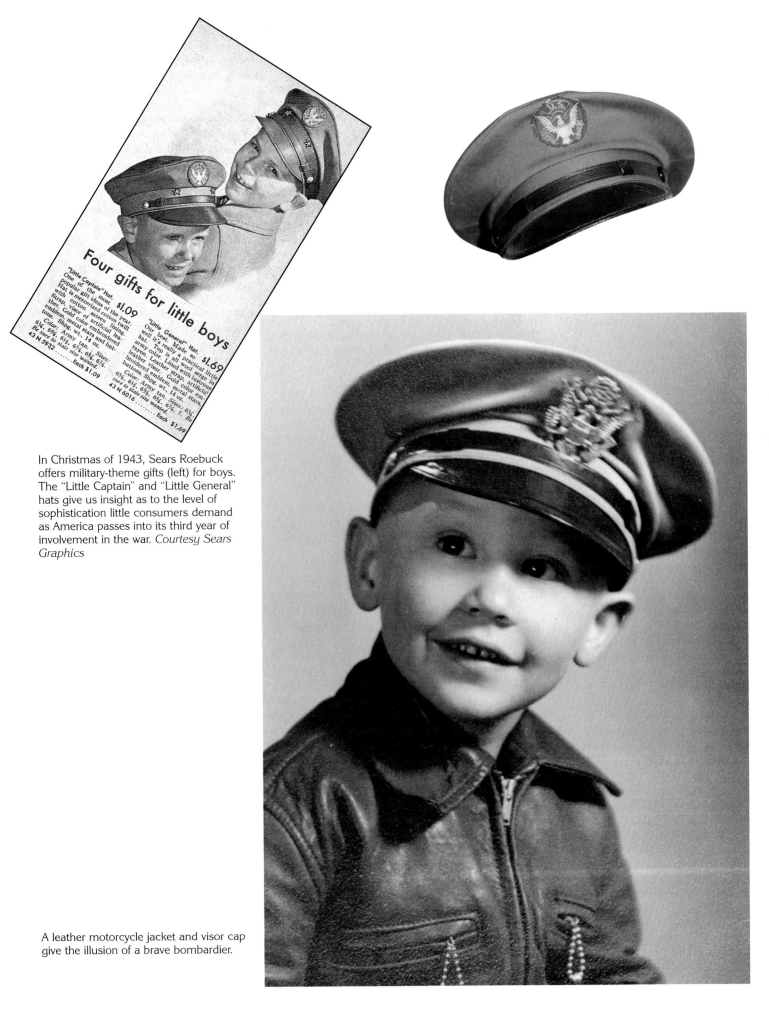

Four gifts for little boys

"Little Captain" Hat. $1.09
One of the most popular gift ideas of the year. Hat is mercerized cotton twill with cotton sateen lining. Strap, visor of artificial leather. Gold color embroidered emblem, metal stars and buttons. Shpg. wt., 14 oz.
Color: Army tan. Sizes: 6¼, 6⅜, 6½, 6⅝, 6¾, 6⅞. Be sure to state size wanted.
43 N 5932 ....Each $1.09

"Little General" Hat. $1.69
Our best. Made so well it's really a practical little hat. Top is all wool serge in army color. Lined with lustrous rayon. Leather strap, artificial leather visor. Gold color embroidered emblem, metal color stars, buttons. Shpg. wt., 14 oz.
Color: Army tan. Sizes: 6¼, 6⅜, 6½, 6⅝, 6¾, 6⅞, 7. Be sure to state size wanted.
43 N 6016 ....Each $1.69

In Christmas of 1943, Sears Roebuck offers military-theme gifts (left) for boys. The "Little Captain" and "Little General" hats give us insight as to the level of sophistication little consumers demand as America passes into its third year of involvement in the war. *Courtesy Sears Graphics*

A leather motorcycle jacket and visor cap give the illusion of a brave bombardier.

131

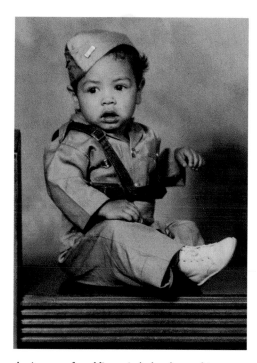

An image of an Hispanic baby dressed in a WWII-style uniform. Photographs of Americans of ethnic background in the patriotic or military genre are seldom found for sale in the collectors' market.

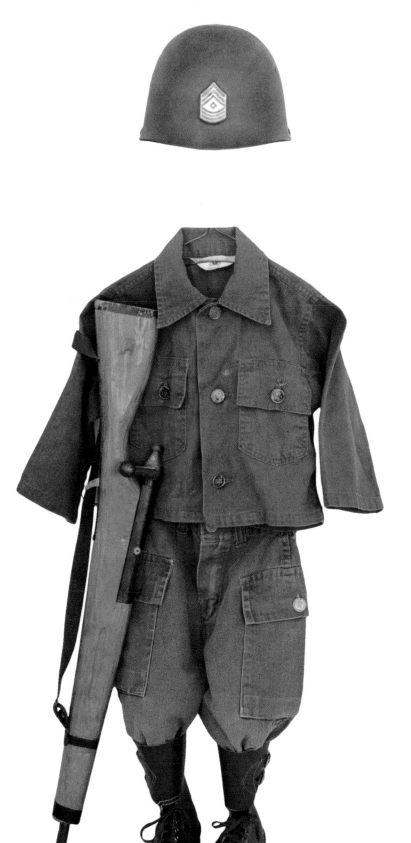

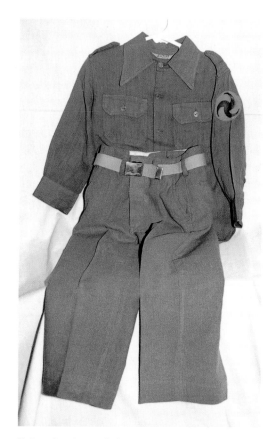

Enlisted-style wool shirt and trousers. The shirt bears a General Headquarters shoulder patch. The U.S. Air Corps used this insignia from 1937 to1941. *Courtesy Kathleen MacDonald Collection*

The herringbone twill uniform bears the maker label of "Fruit of the Loom Sanforized" and military-style buttons. The two buckle boots are marked "Winner Beebe Non-Marking, Tough Wear Toe." The heel is marked "Goal." The plastic helmet dates at least a decade or so later. *Courtesy Debra Allan Collection*

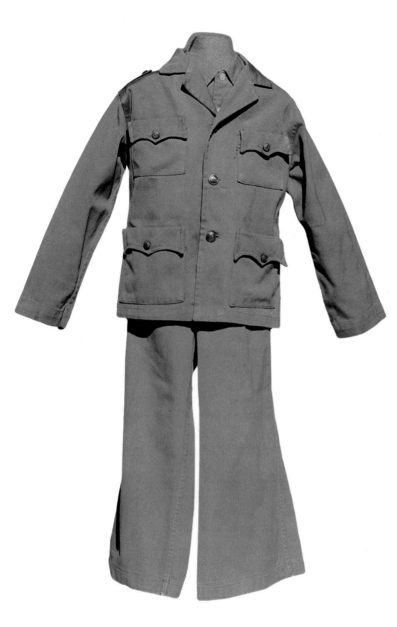

This type of commercially produced khaki Air Force uniform was standard fare for the World War II younger set. This particular example is void of insignia and was almost certainly offered with a cap (not shown). Examples of this type of uniform can be seen in photographs of children wearing similar suits throughout this chapter.

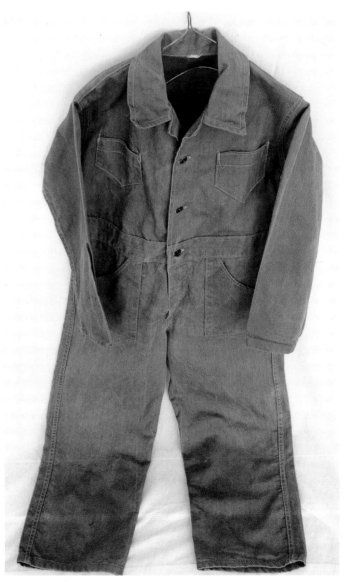

Herringbone twill jumpsuit with civilian buttons. *Courtesy Debra Allan Collection*

Anchors Aweigh!

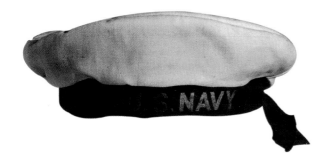

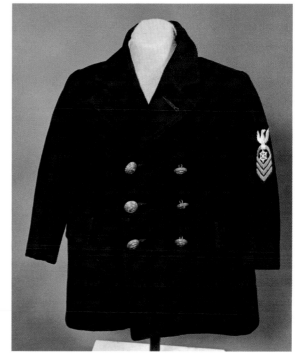

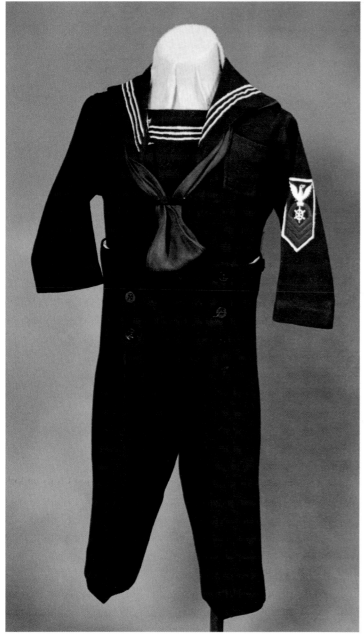

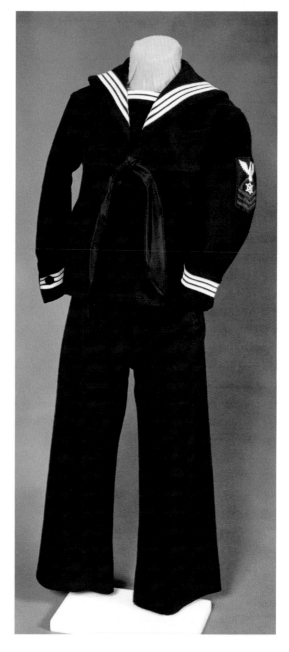

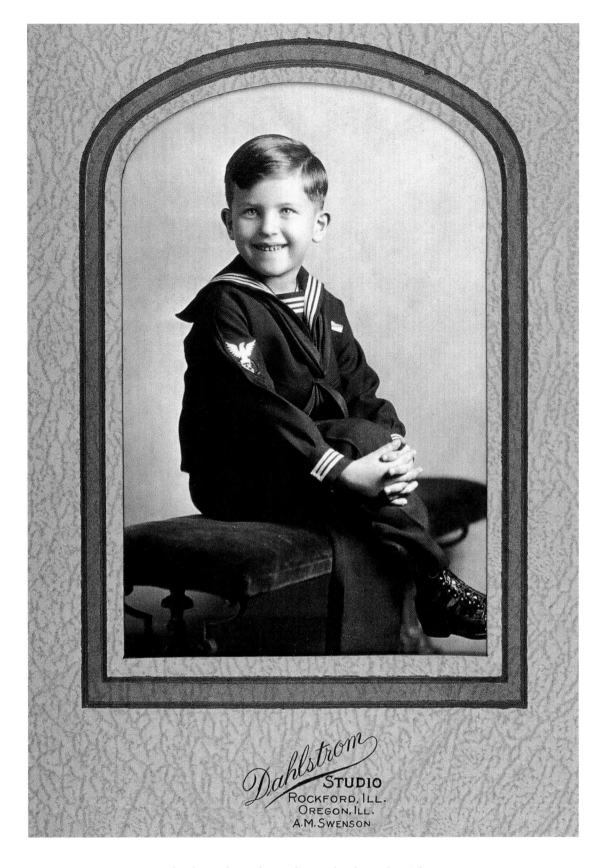

Dahlstrom
STUDIO
ROCKFORD, ILL.
OREGON, ILL.
A.M. SWENSON

Anchors Aweigh my boys, Anchors Aweigh
Farewell to college joys,
We sail at break of day-day-day-day!
Through our last night on shore,
Drink to the foam,
Until we meet once more
Here's wishing you a happy voyage home

World War Overseas...

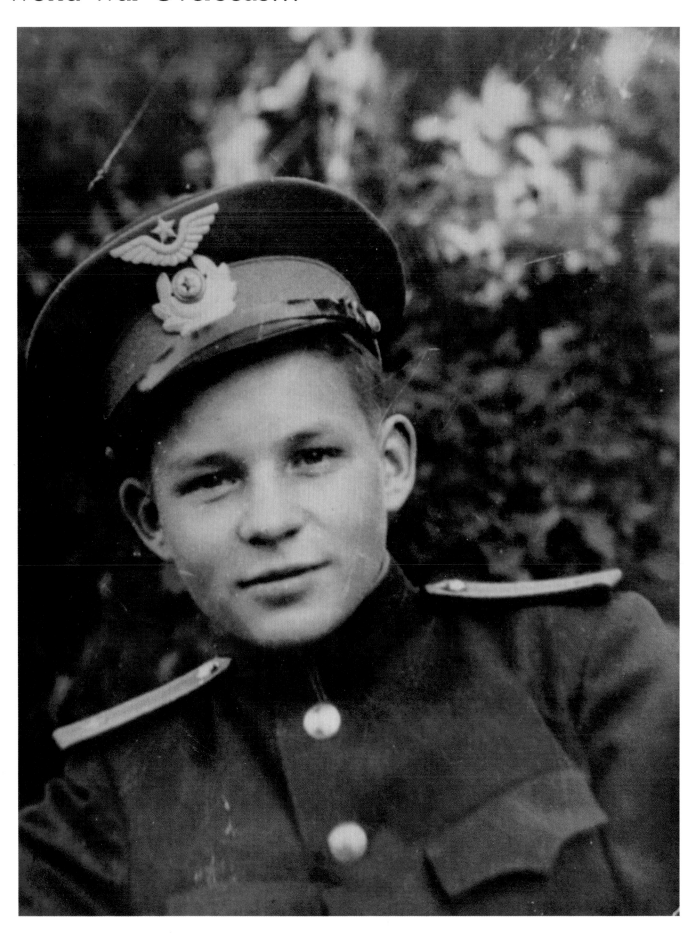

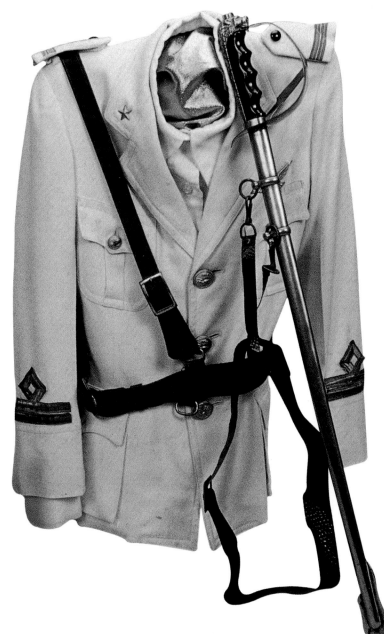

Healthy children orphaned by war were at times picked up and adopted into units by passing troops. Americans followed this practice in the European Theater and the Russians on their own home front, using the term "sons of the regiment" for these boys. They performed a number of tasks for the soldiers such as shining shoes, cleaning weapons, and cleaning up camp. The smartly dressed lad (below) serves an Army unit, while the older boy (opposite page) strikes an engaging balance between adolescent and adult Air Force pilot. The father of the child who wore this uniform (above right) was a member of the Italian Air Force. The uniform is cut for a boy about eight years old and is decorated with gold braid trim, complete with I.A.F. gilt breast pin, Sam Browne belt, and Italian lion-head-motif sword with hanging straps. *Courtesy Marie DiMartini Whittmann Collection. Photo: Charles Jenkins, III*

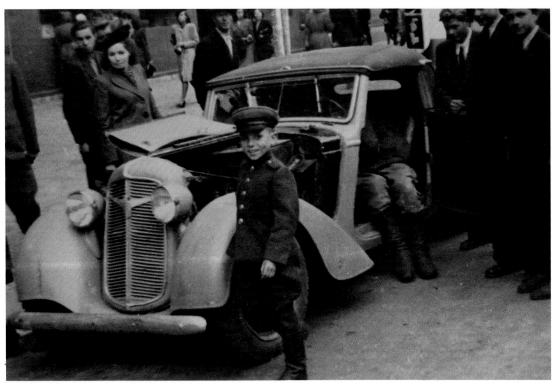

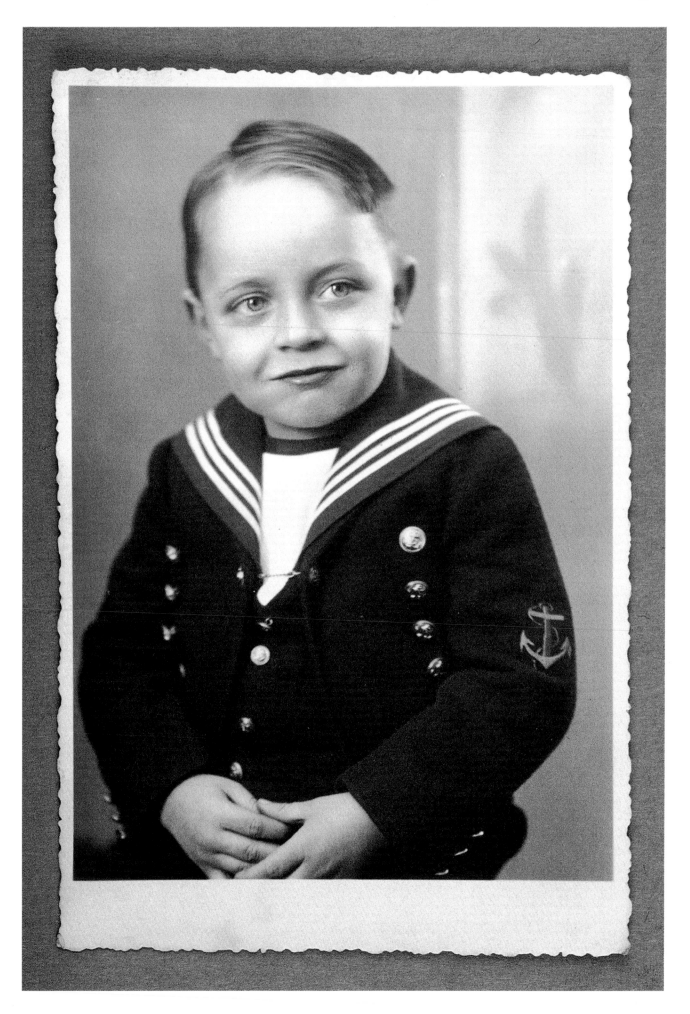

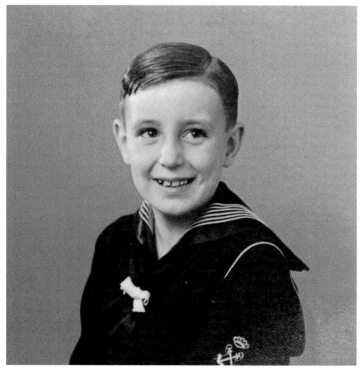

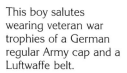

This boy salutes wearing veteran war trophies of a German regular Army cap and a Luftwaffe belt.

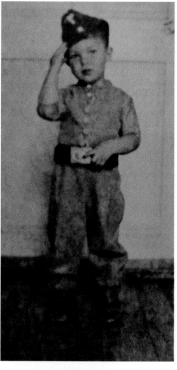

The two boys (above and opposite page) wear two of the many versions of Kriegsmarine (German Navy) uniforms that were as common in Germany during World War II as U.S. Navy-styled suits were a few decades earlier in America. You will see other examples of this same style on the next few pages.

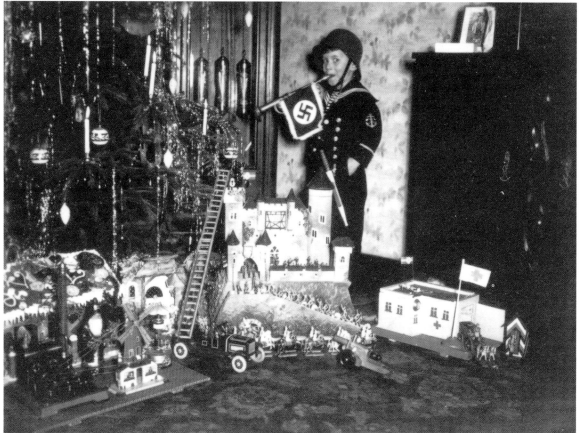

This young Nazi soldier looks quite content with his Christmas haul—a Kriegsmarine suit, Army helmet, dress bayonet, trumpet, and Third Reich trumpet banner. Note the real candles in the Christmas tree. *Courtesy Peter Coleman*

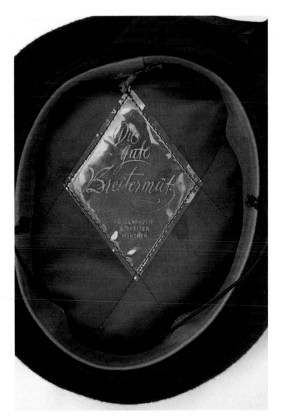

The inside maker label of the hat from the ensemble left. *Courtesy Walter Kanzler*

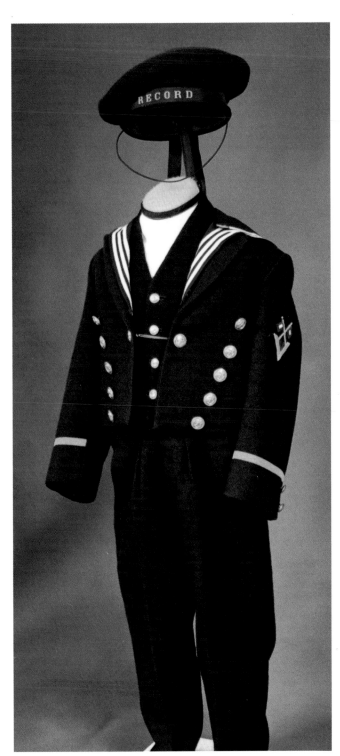

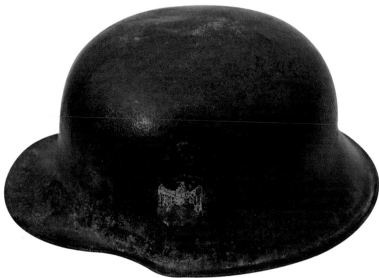

A restored double-decal German Army helmet. The liner is long gone from this example; however, examples that retain the cloth drawstring liner can still occasionally be found.

Courtesy Walter Kanzler

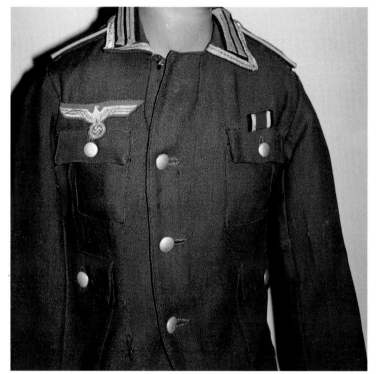

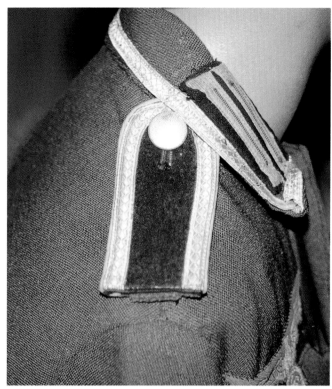

This uniform has qualities of a homemade German fantasy-uniform tunic. The collar insignia is that of an enlisted man. The shoulder straps (above) are that of the lowest-ranking non-commissioned officer, and it includes a standard-issue Army eagle above one pocket and a second-class Iron Cross ribbon on the right. All of these fantastically eclectic qualities make it ideal for a common German boy who wanted to play Army. *Courtesy Peter Coleman*

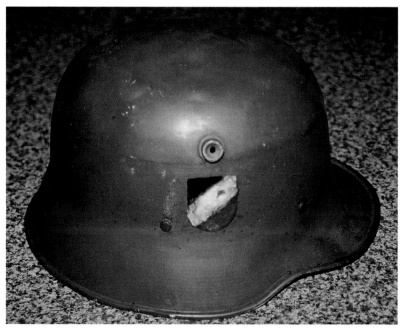

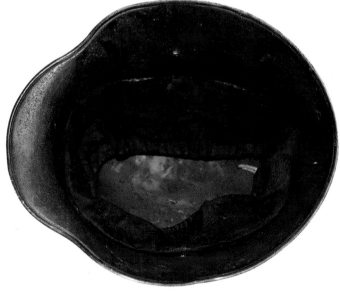

A child's Austrian double-decal helmet. The telltale drawstring liner is seen in the photo above. *Courtesy Peter Coleman*

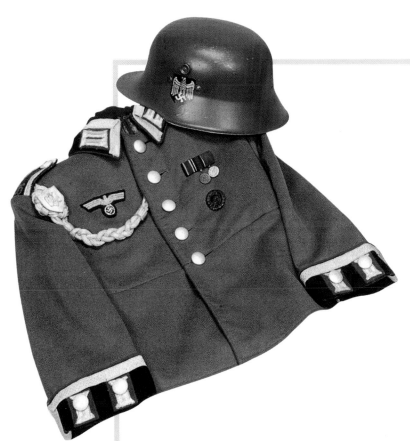

The tiny 3rd Reich Army parade dress tunic is sized for a three-year-old wearer. The uniform is superbly tailored in a soft woolen fabric and piped in red, with *unteroffizer*-style tress decoration. The child's father was an N.C.O. with an artillery regiment. The tunic is outfitted with Shooting Lanyard, Ribbon Bar, and Black Wound Badge, all done in miniature. The accompanying M-35 double-decal helmet is of a child's weight and size. The breast eagle is actually an adult-size cap eagle. *Courtesy Marie DiMartini Whittmann Collection. Photo: Charles Jenkins, III*

The Reichsheer German officer's tunic is an exact replica of the tunic worn by the father of this child. The tunic is sized for a boy of about six years old, reflects fine tailoring, and is fit with slashed side pockets as seen in early-1930s examples prior to the Nazi takeover. The tunic has infantry-designated white piping with sew-in shoulder boards reflecting the rank of *oberleutnant*. *Courtesy Marie DiMartini Whittmann Collection. Photo: Charles Jenkins, III*

The Imperial German Naval waistcoat and accompanying vest are equipped with anchor-embossed gilt-brass buttons. It is sized for a child of about three years old. The child's uniform is lined with silk in the manner of the adult version. The tunic is accompanied by a toy "Naval dirk" produced to realistically duplicate the adult version. The tip of the blade is blunted for safety. *Courtesy Marie DiMartini Whittmann Collection. Photo: Charles Jenkins, III*

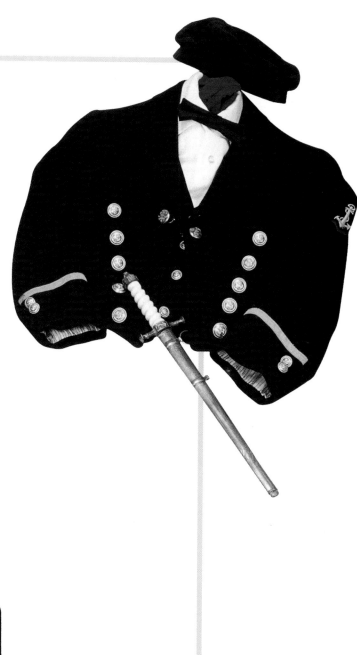

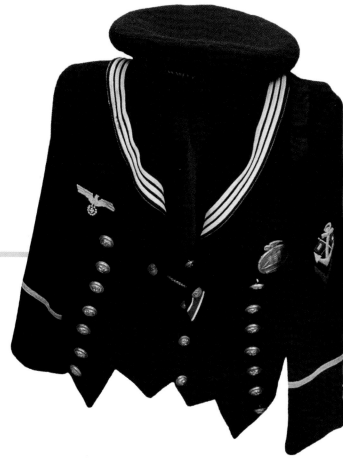

This German Kriegsmarine Naval tunic has a gold-color woven national eagle and swastika sewn to the breast of the tunic, indicating post-1938 vintage. There is an Iron Cross ribbon in the buttonhole, with a Merchant Marine badge at the right breast. The sleeve cloth badge with crossed flags and "V" bar beneath indicate *obersignalmaat* rank. *Courtesy Marie DiMartini Whittmann Collection. Photo: Charles Jenkins, III*

CBI

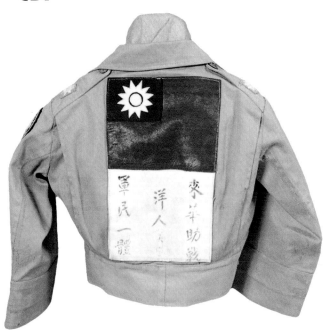

The back view of the "Ike" jacket from the five-piece set, which includes the piece shown, tunic, trousers, belt, and a direct-embroidered OS cap (not shown). The famous "Flying Tigers" made any memorabilia from this theater of operation highly desired back in the States, then and now.

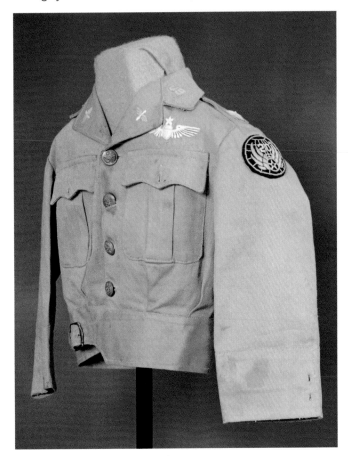

The embroidery on all pieces of this uniform is direct embroidered, including the senior pilot wings on the breast. The 20th Air Force patch is hand-embroidered and scaled to conform to the size of the jacket.

These three pieces, like the others, are direct embroidered. The many tailor shops of Bombay, Calcutta, and Karachi, India, tailored uniforms for a nominal price for servicemen stationed there. The father of the child for whom this outfit was tailored was an Army/Air Force pilot flying mission "over the hump" (over the Himalayas) in the CBI (China, Burma, India) Theater.

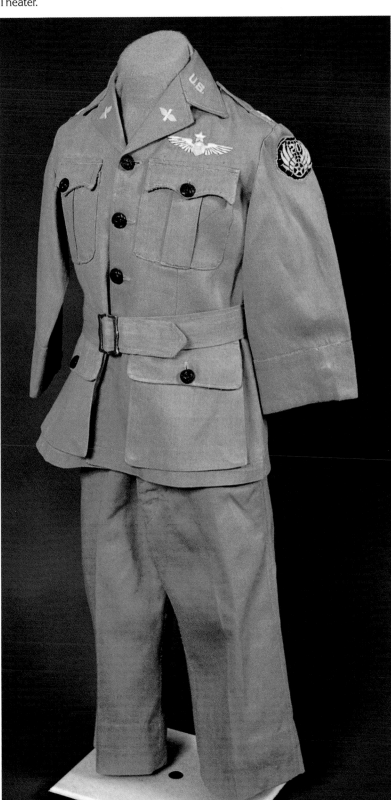

A Primer on Blood Chits

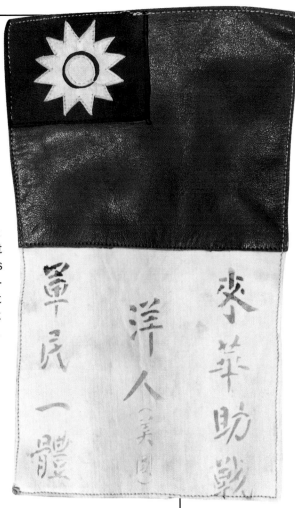

Blood chits have been a part of the kit of military airmen since RFC (Royal Flying Corps) Squadrons on Colonial policing duties in India first received them in 1917, but in no other place and at no other time did blood chits flourish as an art form as they did in the China-Burma-India theater during World War Two.

Foreign military airmen flying against the Japanese in China first received Chinese blood chits in 1938. When the famous American Volunteer Group of the Chinese Air Force (Flying Tigers) reached China in the winter of 1941, they were issued blood chits as well. Originally called Rescue Patches, they were pieces of silk sewn to a cotton backing with the flag of the Republic of China at the top and a message in Chinese printed below it stating, "This foreigner (an American) has come to China to help in the war effort. Soldiers and civilians one and all should rescue and protect him." These were often worn on the backs of flight suits or flight jackets for use in the event that the pilot was forced down and needed to communicate with the local people.

Blood chits were issued to Army/Air Force flying personnel posted to China and India after the United States entered World War Two. Once it was realized that a blood chit sewn to the back of a jacket would hinder an evading airman's concealment from enemy troops, orders were issued that they be sewn only on the inside of jackets, where they could not be seen.

Because of their unique beauty, patches in the form of blood chits remained popular as decorations, even though jackets thus decorated could not be worn on missions. This wonderful child's jacket (far left, opposite page) is an excellent example of that tradition, and the beautiful leather applique patch (close-up, top right) on its back is typical of those produced by local craftsmen for sale to American servicemen. When purchased in the local economy in India in 1944 or 1945, the patch would have cost about three dollars; today it is worth hundreds, and with its authentic period decoration, this jacket for an airman's beloved child might be called priceless.

R.E. Baldwin is a noted expert in the area of miitary aviation escape and evasion, and the author of Last Hope: The Blood Chit Story.

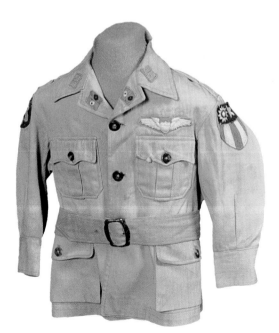

This tunic was probably made late in the war. None of the insignia is direct embroidered, but rather embroidered to cloth of a similar color, then cut out and applied to the tunic separately like patches. The shoulder has a typical CBI cloth patch.

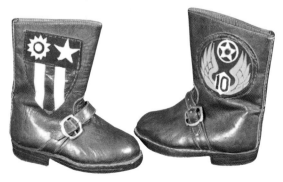

An exceptional pair of all-leather child's boots made with multipiece-construction leather patches of the CBI Theater and a 10th Air Force insignia. These were theater made in India and, like the identical adult version made for servicemen, carry a heavy English influence to the styling. They are made to fit a child of about two to three years old but were never worn.

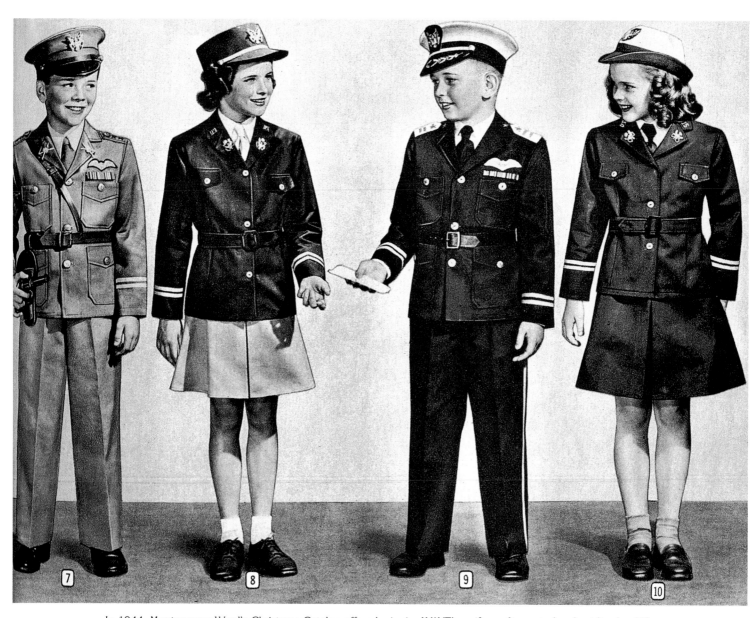

In 1944, Montgomery Ward's Christmas Catalog offered a junior WAVE's uniform. It was to be short-lived; a little more than a year later the war was over. At no other time before or since the war have girls been offered the opportunity to "play war" with costumes of their own. *Courtesy University of Wyoming American Heritage Center*

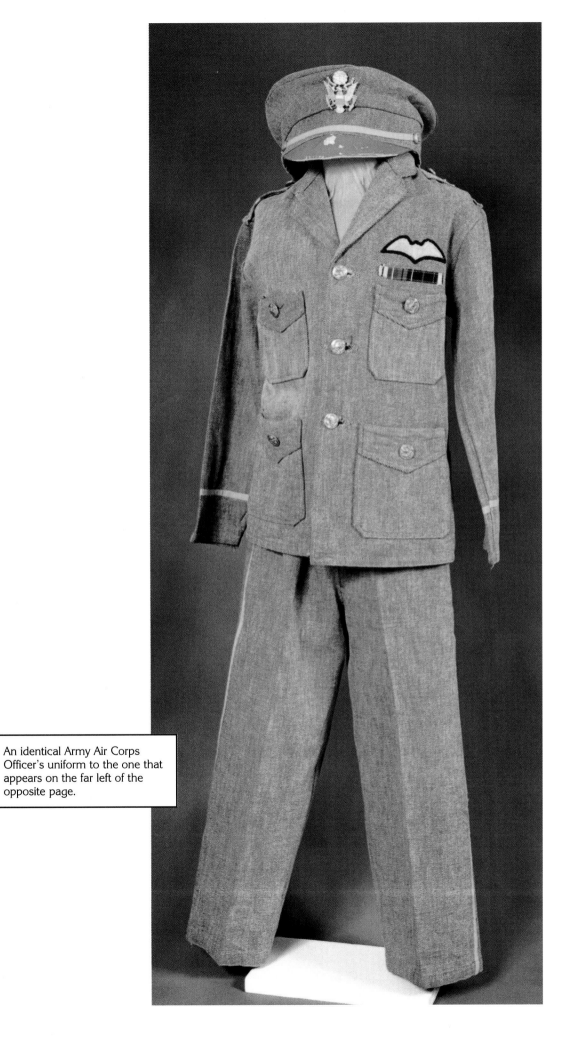

An identical Army Air Corps Officer's uniform to the one that appears on the far left of the opposite page.

Girls Come Front and Center

In 1942, girls were still relegated to non-service-oriented, traditional, subservient roles when it came to play costumes. The war-nurse costume (below) was just a civilian nurse's costume before the war. It does not, in fact, even resemble a military nurse's uniform at all, but if it had to be compared to something from the period, we could match it more to an American Women's Hospital Reserve Corps hospital-aide uniform like the one shown at lower right. *Courtesy George Peterson, NCHS Inc.* Doctor and nurse kits (right) were popular before the war, but once it began, toy companies thought to include military-style armbands in the box, and suddenly regular kits become new and exciting "Army" doctor and nurse kits. Stickers were applied on the box tops to update the kits without the expense of new packaging.

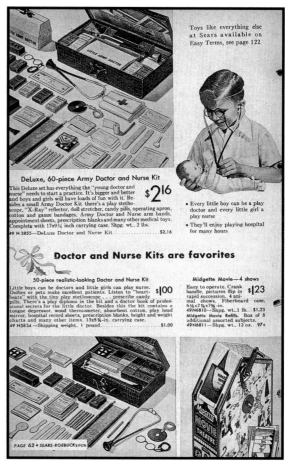

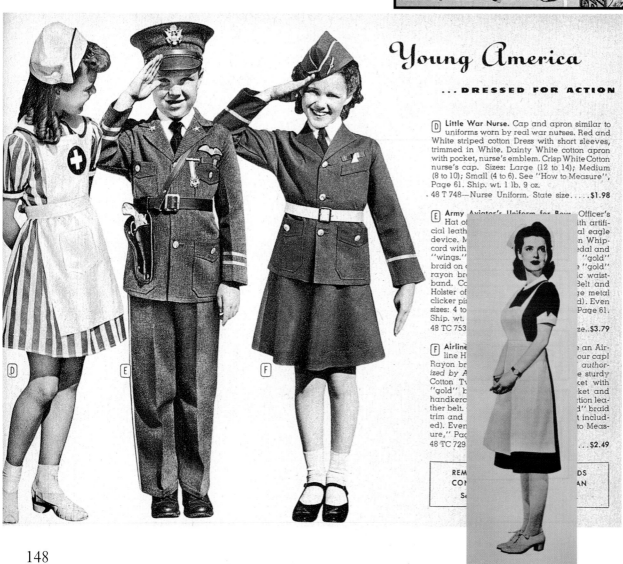

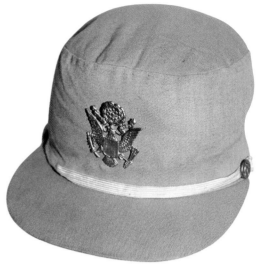

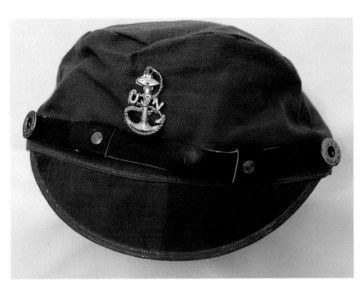

Women's Army Corps uniforms for girls were manufactured by several companies, which accounts for the variation in fabrics, styles, and insignia. The color differences are clear when a page from a wartime regulation-uniform catalog is observed. Dark green is specified for winter, khaki for summer/tropical.

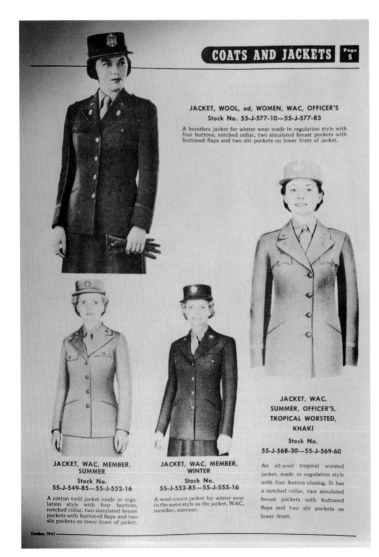

COATS AND JACKETS Page 5

JACKET, WOOL, od, WOMEN, WAC, OFFICER'S
Stock No. 55-J-577-10—55-J-577-83

A barathea jacket for winter wear made in regulation style with four buttons, notched collar, two simulated breast pockets with buttoned flaps and two slit pockets on lower front of jacket.

JACKET, WAC, SUMMER, OFFICER'S, TROPICAL WORSTED, KHAKI
Stock No. 55-J-568-30—55-J-569-60

An all-wool tropical worsted jacket, made in regulation style with four button closing. It has a notched collar, two simulated breast pockets with buttoned flaps and two slit pockets on lower front.

JACKET, WAC, MEMBER, SUMMER
Stock No. 55-J-549-85—55-J-552-16

A cotton twill jacket made in regulation style with four buttons, notched collar, two simulated breast pockets with buttoned flaps and two slit pockets on lower front of jacket.

JACKET, WAC, MEMBER, WINTER
Stock No. 55-J-552-85—55-J-555-16

A wool covert jacket for winter wear in the same style as the jacket, WAC, member, summer.

October, 1943

Courtesy George Peterson, NCHS Inc.

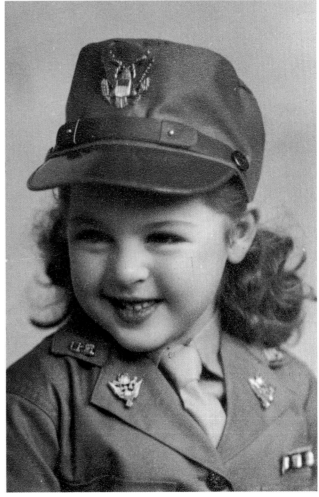

This little darling is the spitting image of her adult counterpart in the photo to the left.

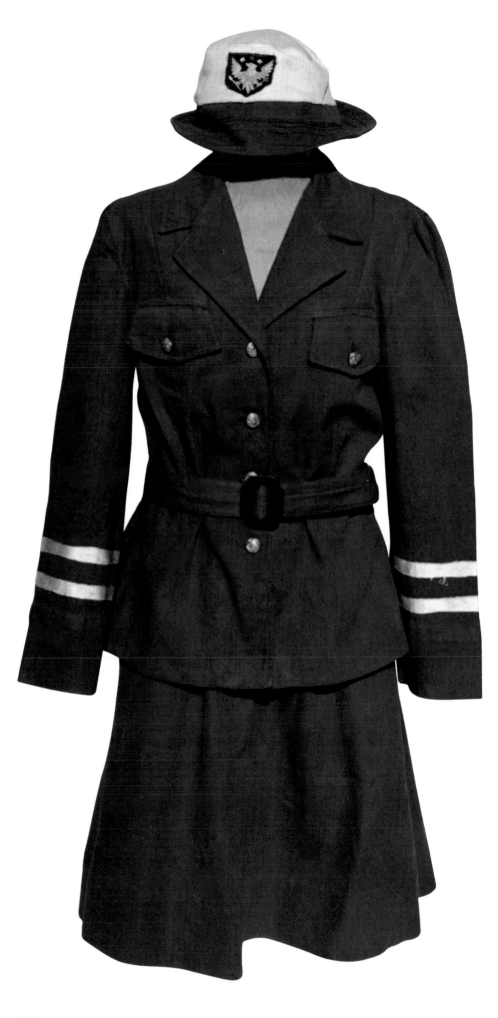

A version of the 1944 Ward catalog offered junior WAVE outfits. This one has the complicated multipiece-construction hat and is styled most closely to the adult version.

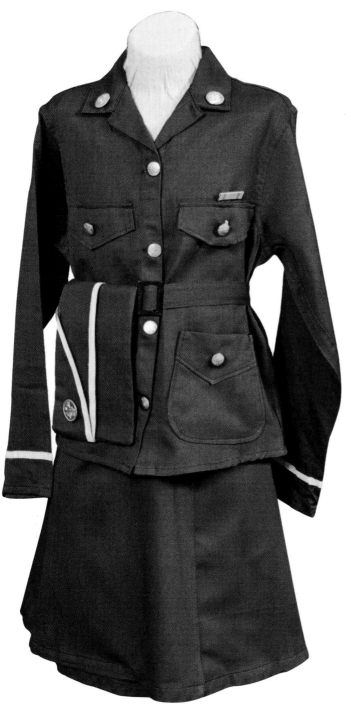

Truth be known, this junior WAVE's costume was an "Airplane Hostess Uniform" (page 148) converted to accommodate wartime demand for girls' junior WAVE costumes. By replacing the white belt with a blue belt and adding a few military-style buttons to the pockets, a "U.S." collar insignia, and a National Defense ribbon bar, the transformation is complete, helping out the manufacturer twofold—a quintessential stroke of American ingenuity.

Yet another junior WAVE. This version has a dark hat and terrific fantasy sleeve patch. *Courtesy Kathleen MacDonald Collection.*

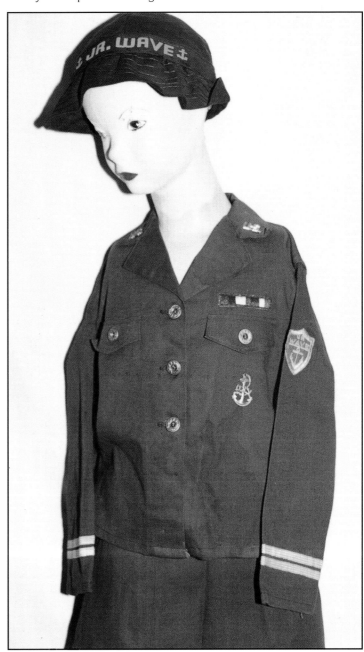

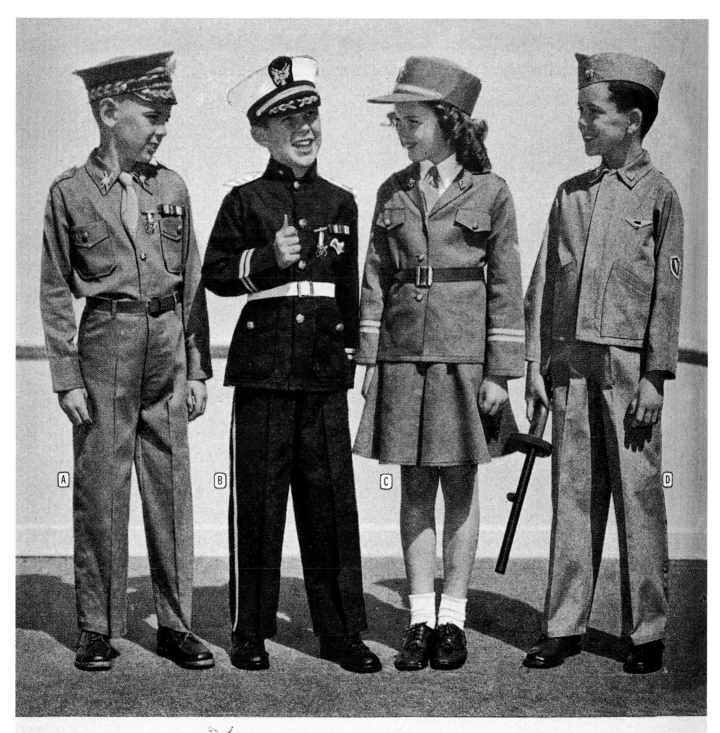

Play clothes in military styling

A GENERALS' UNIFORM FOR BOYS. Strong Cotton Drill tuck-in Shirt and Trousers. Officer's medal, "gold" infantry insignia, belt and tie are included. Embroidered General's Cap has metal eagle. EVEN SIZES: 4 to 12 yrs. *State Size.* See "How to Measure," Page 93.
48 X 769—Ship. wt. 2 lbs. 8 oz.............$3.10

B NAVAL OFFICERS' UNIFORM FOR BOYS. Blue Cotton Twill, white belt. Trousers have "gold" braid, elastic waistband. Embroidered Navy Officer's Cap, metal eagle. "Wings" and officer's medal. EVEN SIZES: 4 to 12 yrs. *State Size.* See "How to Measure," opposite page.
48 X 770—Ship. wt. 2 lbs. 8 oz.............$3.10

C LITTLE GIRLS' "WAC" UNIFORM. Light-weight Cotton Twill. Unlined Jacket is belted, has mock pockets. Flare skirt with kick-pleat in front. WAC cap carries metal emblem. Blouse, tie not included. EVEN SIZES: 4 to 14 yrs. *State size.* See "How to Measure," opposite page.
48 X 773—Ship. wt. 2 lbs. 8 oz.............$2.89

D JR. COMMANDO. Field Jacket-Overall outfit with Overseas Cap. A fine suit, Zelan treated (water-repellent) Olive Drab Cotton, pre-shrunk, washable. Jacket has deep pockets, buckle hip straps. Overall-top trousers. EVEN SIZES: 4 to 10 yrs. See "How to Measure," Page 93.
48 X 804—*State size.* Ship. wt. 2 lbs......$3.79

E WOOD DRILL RIFLE. Realistic dummy Rifle and Manual of Infantry Drill Regulations. Of polished hardwood, nicely turned and finished with sturdy carrying sling so boy can practice actual firing positions. Dummy pump action unit. Overall length about 37 in. *Mailable.*
48 T 777—Ship. wt. 2 lbs. 4 oz. $1.63

F CHATTERMATIC "SUB MACHINE" GUN. Turning crank makes a rat-a-tat. Walnut finished stock, red cylindrical "magazine," black wood barrel and grip. Length 24 inches. Made by the manufacturers of the real Daisy Air Rifle. Better finish than most guns at this price.
48 X 772—Ship. wt. 1 lb. *Mailable*..........84c

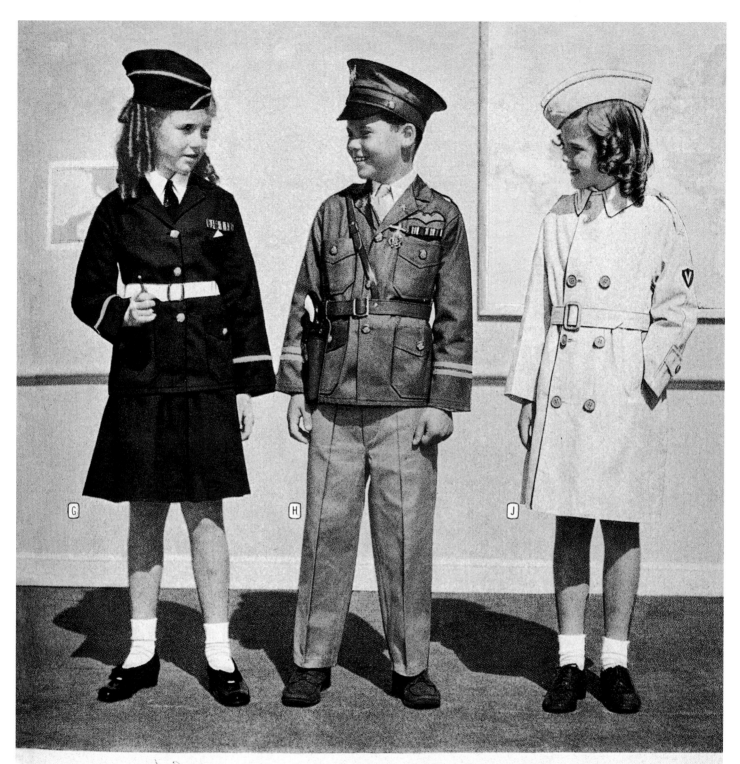

Service uniforms for active juniors

G AIRPLANE HOSTESS UNIFORM FOR GIRLS. Blue Cotton Twill jacket has "gold" braid trim. White belt, flared skirt. (Blouse, tie, not included.) Overseas cap with metal "Wings" authorized by American Airlines. EVEN SIZES: 4 to 14 yrs. State size. Read "How to Measure."
48 T 733—Ship. wt. 2 lbs. 2 oz.............$2.49

HOW TO MEASURE FOR GIRLS' AND BOYS' OUTFITS. Order coat and pants of outfit in same size. Be sure outfit is listed in size you order.

Order size	4	6	8	10	12	14
If chest is	23 in.	24½	26	27½	29	30½
If waist is	23 in.	23½	24	25	26	26½

H ARMY AIR CORPS OFFICERS' UNIFORM FOR BOYS. Well tailored, of heavy Cotton Twill—Jacket Khaki color, pants lighter Tan. Officers' hat has metal insignia. Sam Browne belt and holster of split leather. Wood-plastic toy pistol. EVEN SIZES: 4 to 12 yrs. See "How to Measure."
48 T 734—State size. Ship. wt. 3 lbs.......$4.69

J GIRLS' MILITARY RAINCOAT AND CAP. Light tan double breasted trench coat of sturdy Impregnole-finish (rain-resistant) Cotton Drill. Deep pockets; colorful plaid cotton flannel lining. Matching cotton drill Overseas Cap. EVEN SIZES: 4 to 12 yrs. State size. See "How to Measure."
48 T 788—Ship. wt. 3 lbs. 8 oz.............$4.98

K BOYS' WOOD TOMMY GUN. Gives a loud rat-a-tat-tat—when you slide forward grip along the barrel. Walnut-finished wood play gun, 30 in. long, with 6-in. "bullet cylinder."
48 T 822—Ship. wt. 1 lb. 12 oz............$1.98

L CHROME PLATED METAL BATON. Professional weight and balance. Spiral grip. 28 in. long. ¾-in. shaft. Wood ball and tip. Act. wt. 13 oz.
51 X 2171—Ship. wt. 1 lb. 4 oz............$1.95

M SILVER COLORED HARDWOOD BATON. 28½ in. long ¾-in. shaft. Act. wt. 7 oz. Instructions.
51 X 2165—Ship. wt. 1 lb.................69c

See Baton Twirling Books in General Catalog.

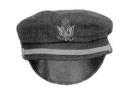

The Women's Army Auxiliary Corps (WAAC) was founded on March 14, 1942. On September 30, 1943, WAAC became U.S. WAC, (Women's Army Corps), and at its peak in April 1945, the WACs had 99,000 women in uniform, giving girls of the era a role model dressed in a regulation uniform of the U.S. Armed Forces.

Well-loved and worn, this early junior WAC outfit (left) carries the more obscure WAAC sleeve insignia. The sturdily constructed hat has a stenciled hat device and retains the blouse, which was normally sold separately. *Courtesy Kathleen MacDonald Collection*

This junior WAC outfit (lower left) is missing the sleeve patch, or it was never put on at the factory. High demand sometimes dictated that costumes leave with missing or substituted insignia, as seen in the example below. The Army eagle lapel and hat devices have been substituted with Navy, and the "U.S." collar devices are non-existent, a mere technicality, I'm sure, for the lucky girl who wore it.

Some early manufacturers also offered a WAC purse (not shown) in WAC ensembles. These crudely cut and fashioned brown leatherette purses are recognized by their rough and exposed edges. Most companies phased them out quickly due to high demand for the uniforms and production costs.

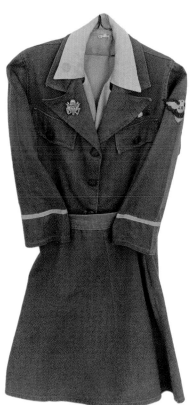

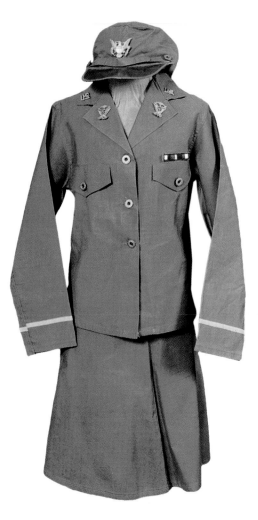

Opposite page:
The boy Campbell's Kid gets in on the act by donning a Montana Peak campaign hat and taking aim at the enemy. He's assigned to "Company C," of course.

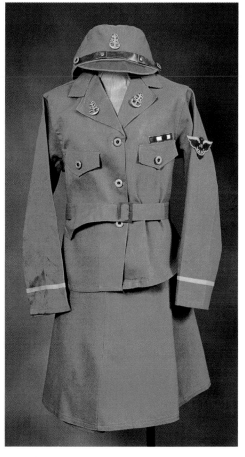

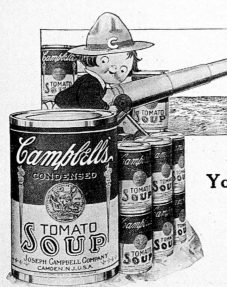

Your "first line of defence"—

Good food and good digestion! These are the first and most important protection for all your physical resources.

The enemies of robust health have no chance even to *land* on your constitution when its "coast-line" is properly defended. And there isn't a defence in the whole line which gives you better protective service than

Campbell's Tomato Soup

It not only supplies effectual nourishment in itself, but it tones and invigorates the appetite and the digestive powers so that you gain increased nutrition from other foods.

No doubt you know this popular Campbell's Soup as an attractive dinner-course. You know it is delicious and inviting. But do you realize its value as a high-efficiency food-product? Do you realize that such a wholesome soup eaten regularly with meals acts as a constant reinforcement of health and vitality?

Why wouldn't this nourishing Campbell "kind" be fine for dinner today?

21 kinds   **10c a can**

Campbell's Soups

LOOK FOR THE RED-AND-WHITE LABEL

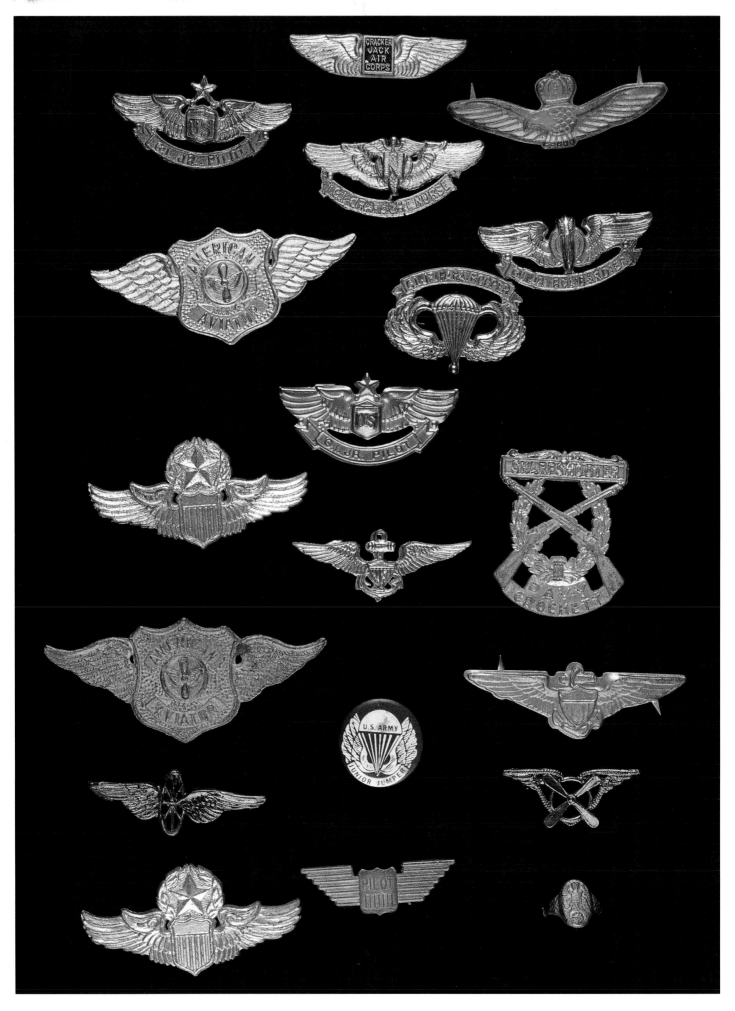

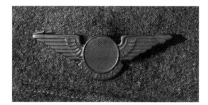

An unidentified Junior Pilot wing. Junior Pilot wings have maintained almost constant popularity from the early days of aviation to the present.

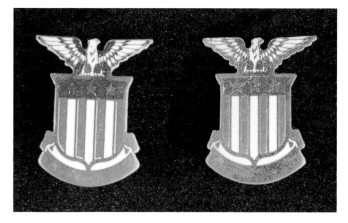

A pair of painted collar devices for a child's uniform.

Opposite:
A grouping of insignia made especially for children.

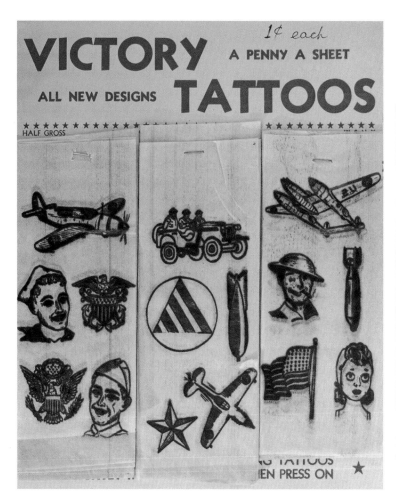

Several designs of "Victory Tattoos" were offered during the war. Some featured "All Navy" or "All Air Force" designs. This one is of particular interest since it features "Rosie the Riveter" in her famous kerchief and netted hairstyle. In the late 1990s a cache of NOS tattoo store cards was found in an old toy warehouse, and subsequently these cards are easily found to add to one's collection.

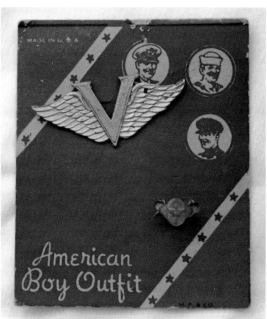

"American Boy Outfits" were not really "outfits" at all, but rather just what you see still intact on the original card. A fantasy "V" wing and military-style ring.

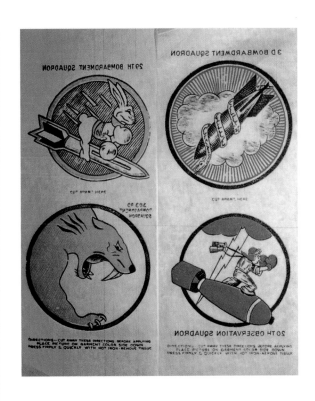

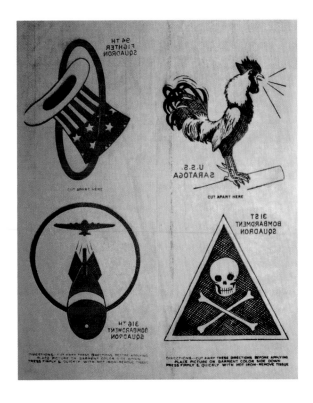

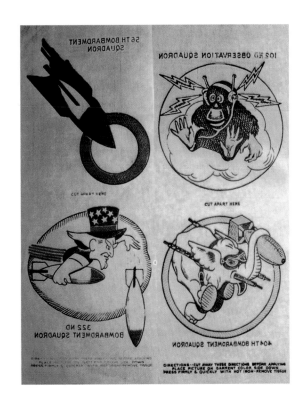

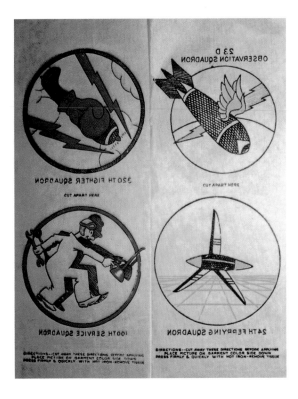

Iron-on transfers (shown in downside, reverse) of genuine fighter and bombardment squadrons were available as product premiums. Many intriguing and patriotic styles of famous squadrons were offered to keep youngsters' interest piqued.

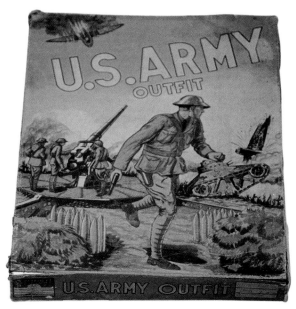

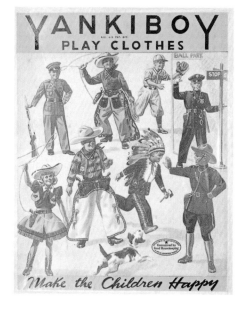

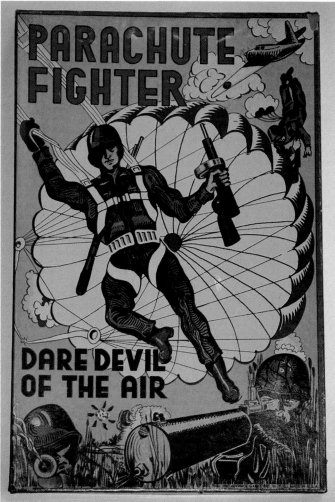

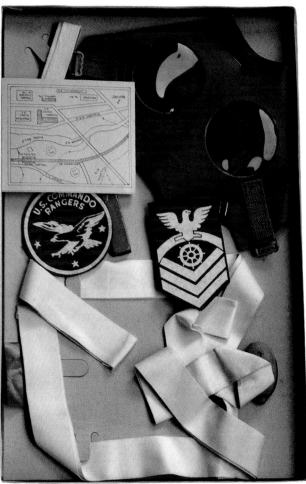

Costumes were sold in boxes that featured elaborate box art, which made the thrill of fantasy soldiering much more real. The box art for the "Army Outfit" (top left) looks at first as if it may have been from WWI, but the closed-cockpit plane in the top left corner dates it closer to WWII. The copyright on the box is 1941. *Courtesy Jack Matthews Collection*

"Yankiboy Play Clothes" (top right) offers a variety of period heroes on the top of its versatile box. The manufacturer prominently displays the "Good Housekeeping Seal of Approval," a sign of quality to American moms who had the daunting task of being the ultimate "smart consumers" during the war. The "Parachute Fighter" costume (above) leaves a little to be desired when the contents are revealed. Note the mixing of Army and Navy insignia in the ensemble, a common practice in children's military-theme toys. *Courtesy Jack Matthews Collection*

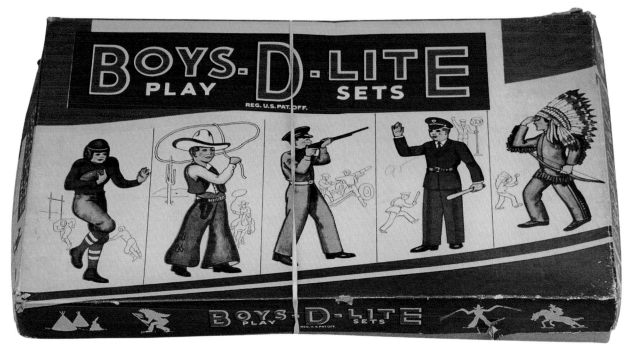

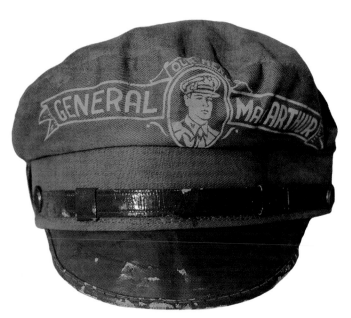

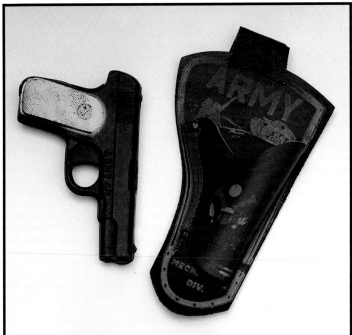

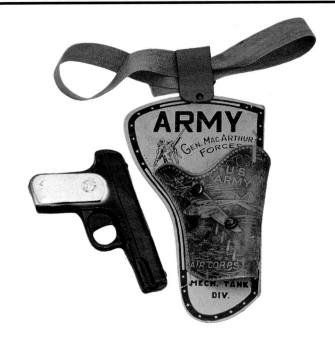

Few military figures during WWII were more beloved by the American public than General Douglas MacArthur. His name and image were brazenly used by anyone who wanted to make a buck during the war, toy manufactures notwithstanding, as evidenced by a few examples shown here.

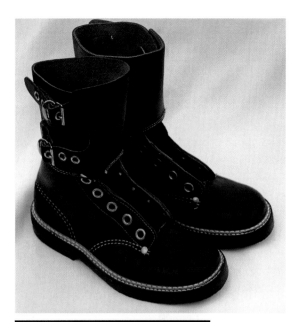

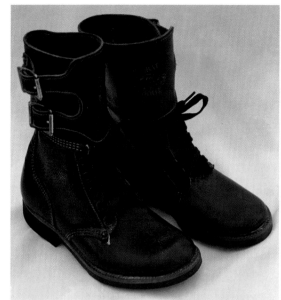

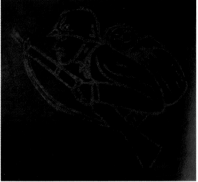

Two-buckle G.I.-style boots were a hot commodity for young would-be commandos. They are easily identified by the military-theme illustrations on the buckle flaps. After the war ended, a surplus of boots remained. These remaining boots were sold without the illustrations, or the theme was changed to reflect interests of the post-war era. I recently observed a new old stock pair with a (non-military) motorcycle rider on the flap at a collectibles show.

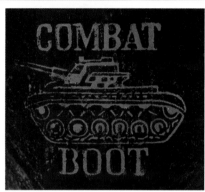

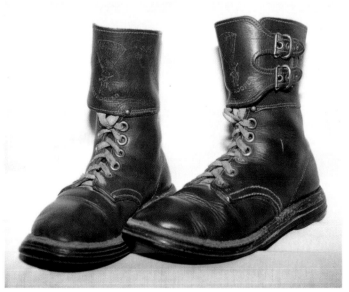

This well-loved pair has "Jr. Paratrooper" beneath the parachutist illustration stenciled on the buckle flap.

A pair of "Stone Mountain" brand brown boots that could easily be mistaken for kids' combat boots to the novice collector. Boys of this era wore this style of shoe for everyday wear, which should not be confused with those clearly manufactured for playing soldier.

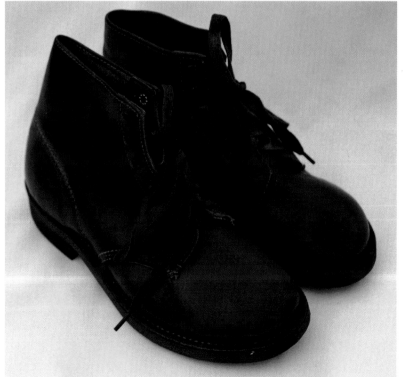

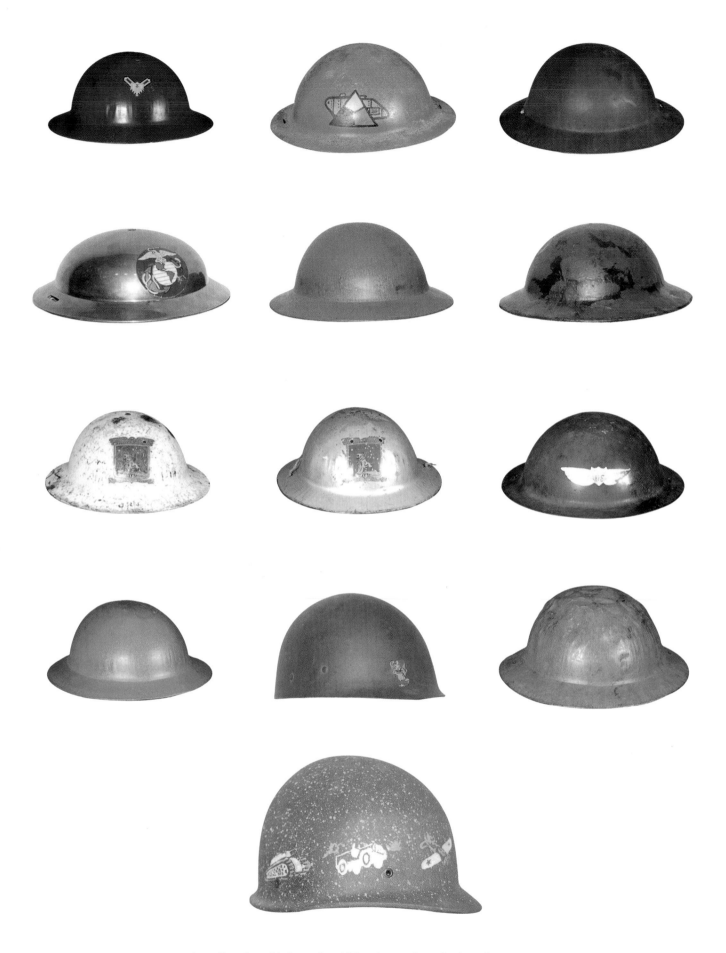

A medley of steel helmets for children in a variety of paint schemes
from the collections of Kathleen MacDonald and the author.

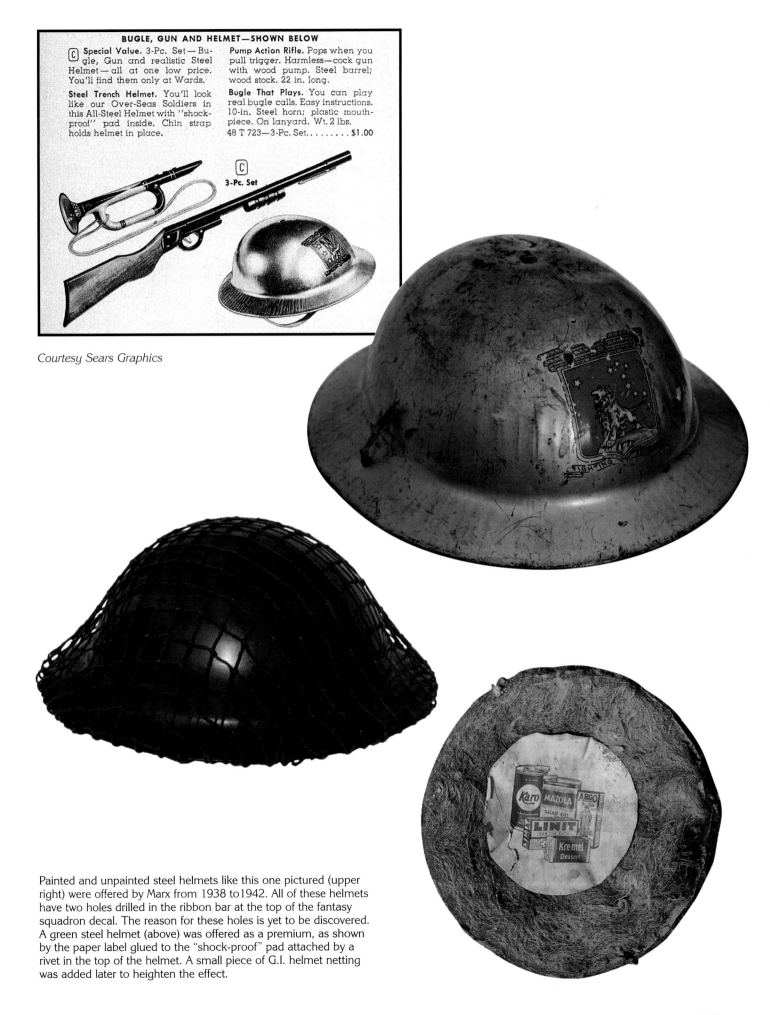

Courtesy Sears Graphics

Painted and unpainted steel helmets like this one pictured (upper right) were offered by Marx from 1938 to 1942. All of these helmets have two holes drilled in the ribbon bar at the top of the fantasy squadron decal. The reason for these holes is yet to be discovered. A green steel helmet (above) was offered as a premium, as shown by the paper label glued to the "shock-proof" pad attached by a rivet in the top of the helmet. A small piece of G.I. helmet netting was added later to heighten the effect.

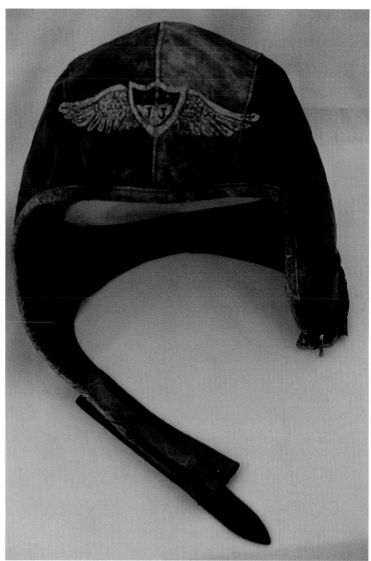

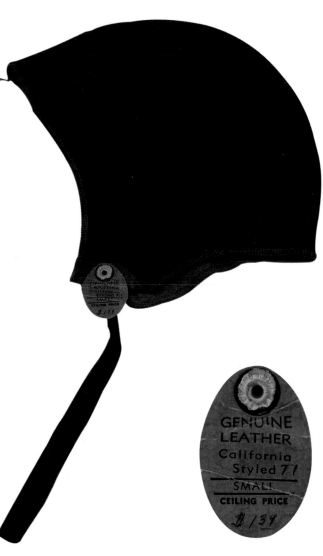

An adult leather flying helmet has been cut and resized for a child. A beautiful wing has been painted on the front with the child's initials.

A WWII-era child's NOS (new old stock) felt-lined leather flying helmet retains its original price tag.

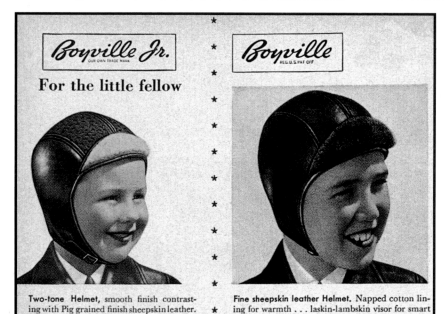

Left:
As troops returned home in 1945, interest in the military waned. Leather helmet-style hats advertised as "aviators' helmets" before and during the war suddenly reverted to utilitarian snow hats. *Courtesy Sears Graphics*

Opposite page photos:
All four of these wartime portraits were taken by the same photographic studio in Inglewood, California. *Courtesy Bob Chatt, Vintage Productions, Huntington Beach, California and Mike Constable*

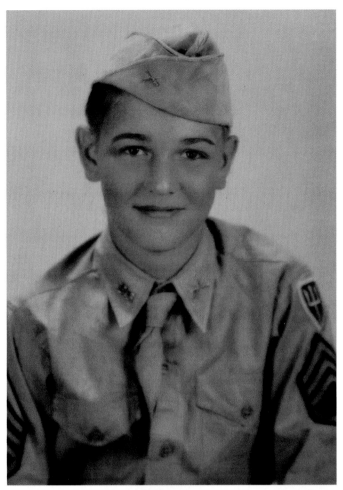

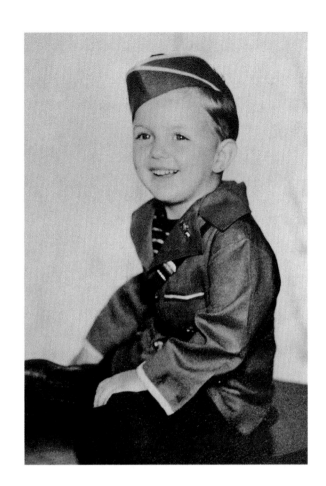

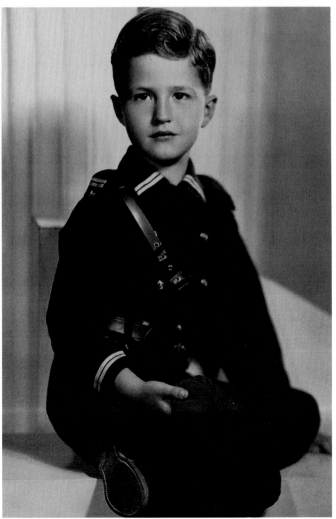

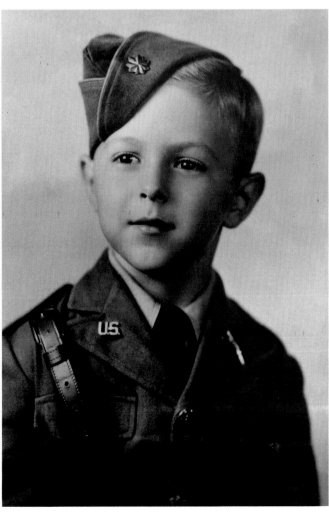

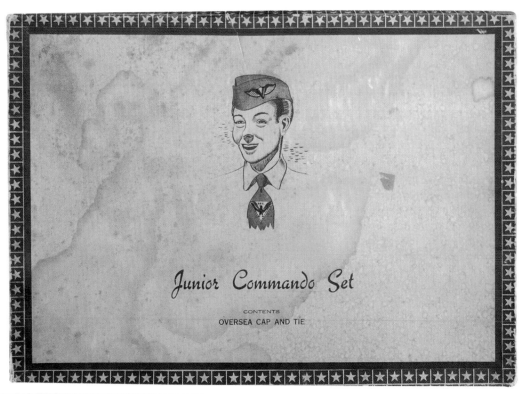

Junior Commando Set

CONTENTS
OVERSEA CAP AND TIE

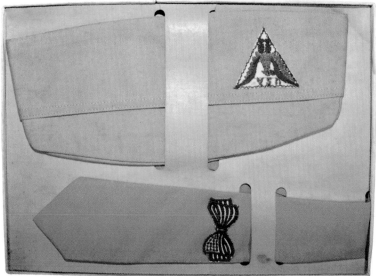

"Junior" anything was a buzz word during WWII for kids wanting to be everything from commandos to WACs. A Junior Commando tie and OS cap gift set (above and right). A group photo of "Alexander and Jr. Commandos" (below). I would guess it's safe to assume Alexander is the boy dressed in white. Circa February 1942.

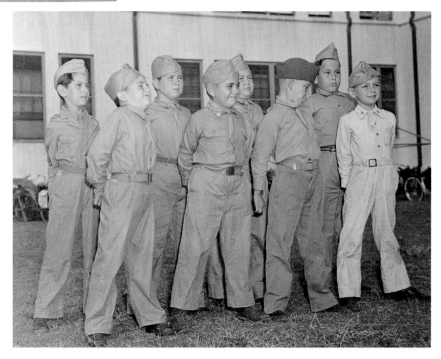

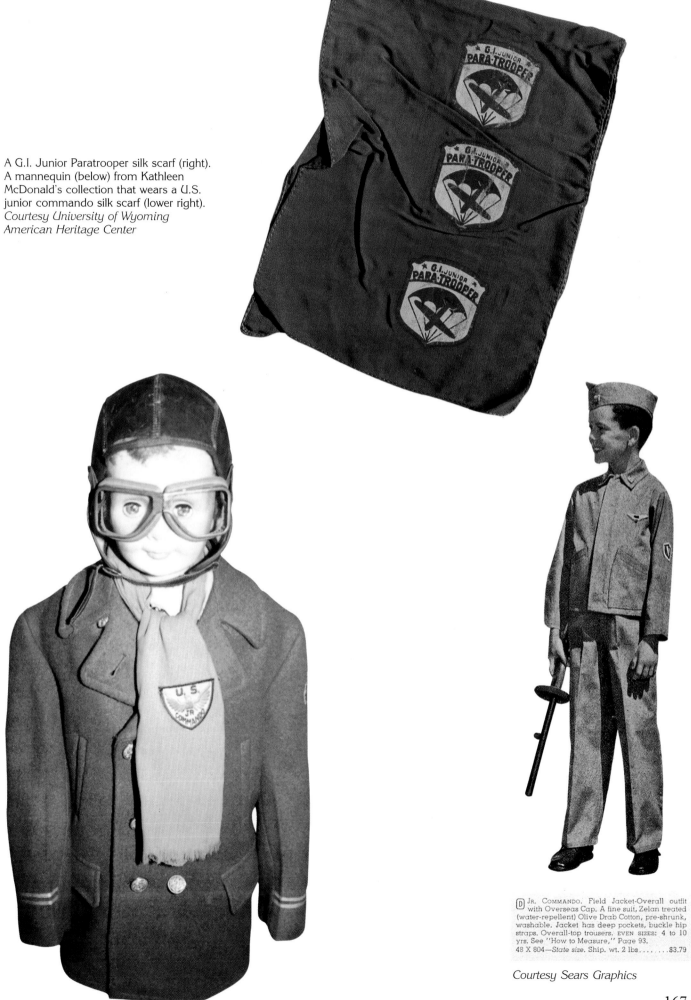

A G.I. Junior Paratrooper silk scarf (right). A mannequin (below) from Kathleen McDonald's collection that wears a U.S. junior commando silk scarf (lower right). *Courtesy University of Wyoming American Heritage Center*

D JR. COMMANDO. Field Jacket-Overall outfit with Overseas Cap. A fine suit, Zelan treated (water-repellent) Olive Drab Cotton, pre-shrunk, washable. Jacket has deep pockets, buckle hip straps. Overall-top trousers. EVEN SIZES: 4 to 10 yrs. See "How to Measure," Page 93. 48 X 804—*State size.* Ship. wt. 2 lbs........$3.79

Courtesy Sears Graphics

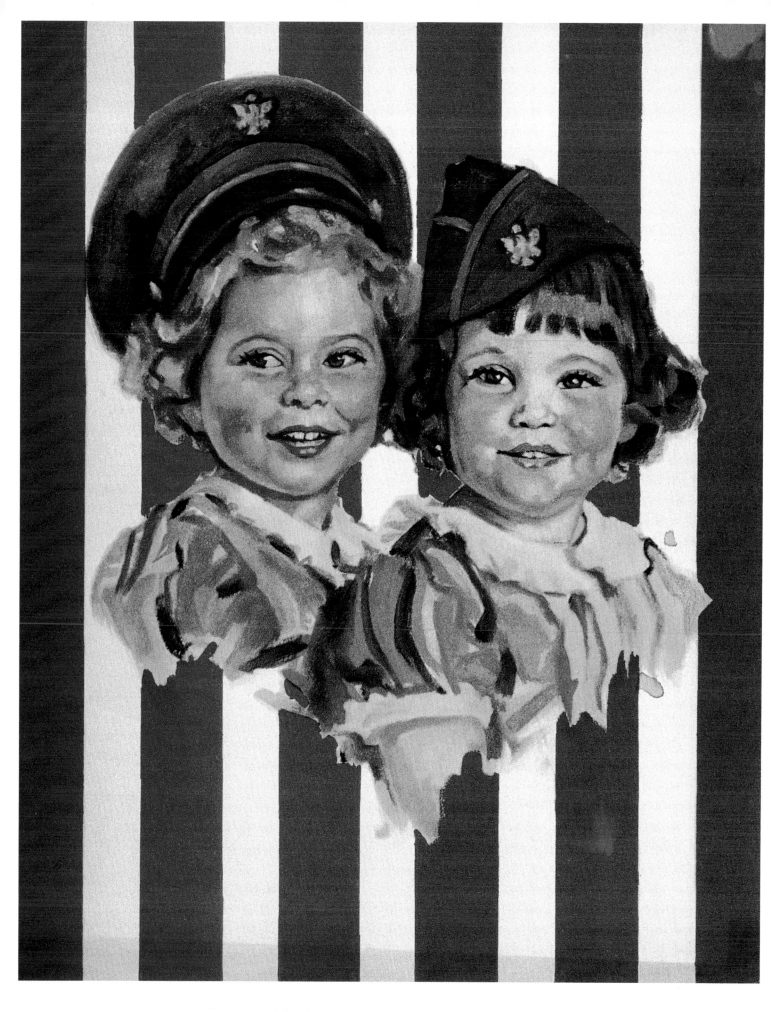

168

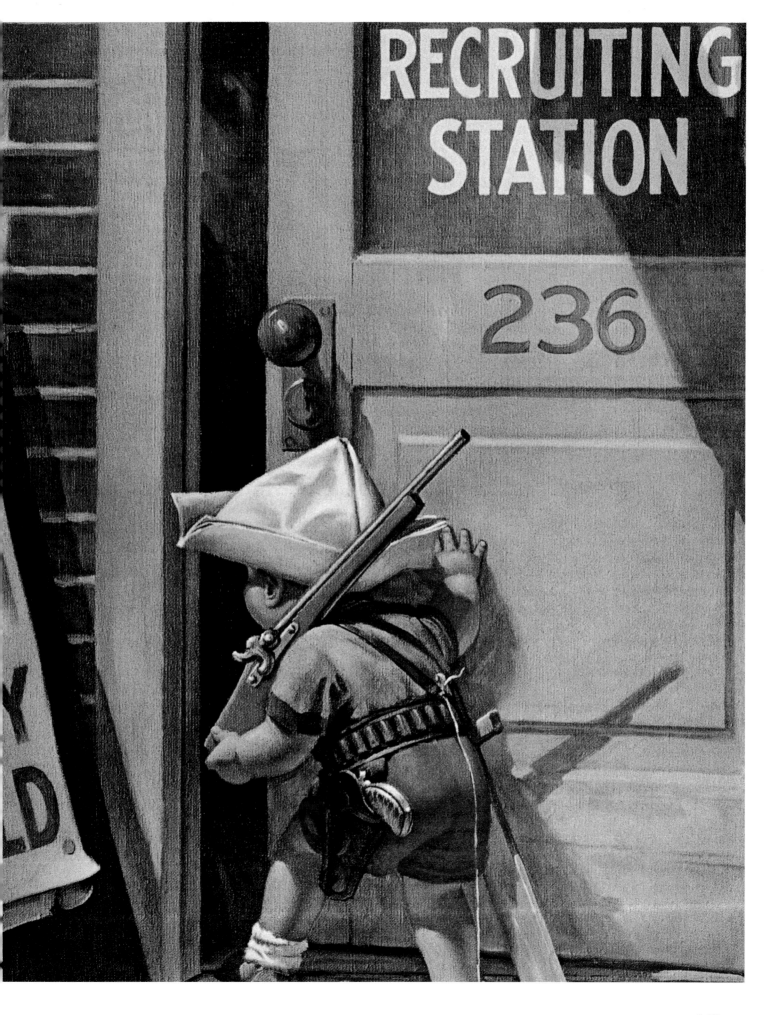

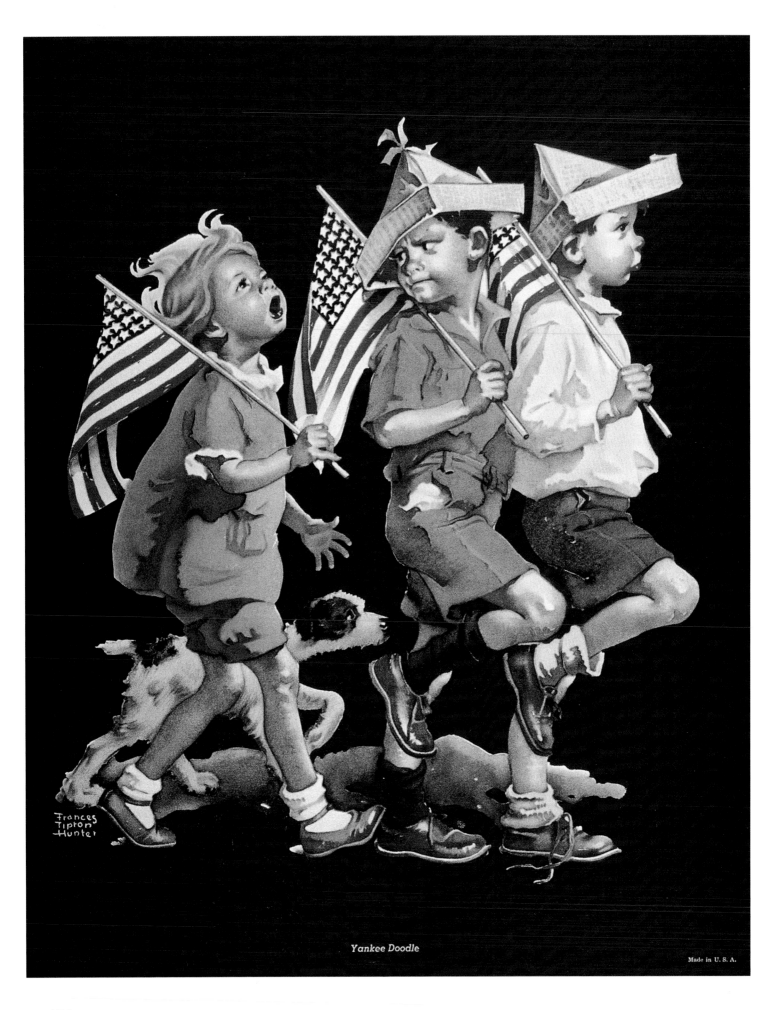

Yankee Doodle

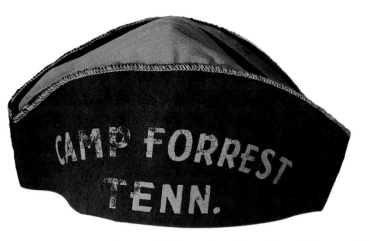
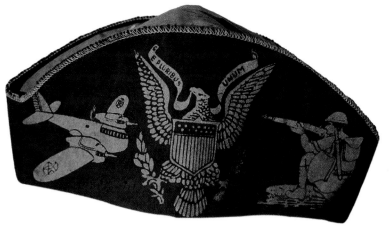

A souvenir OS cap from Camp Forrest, Tennessee. Many bases around the country sold similar hats to recruits who sent them home to family and friends.

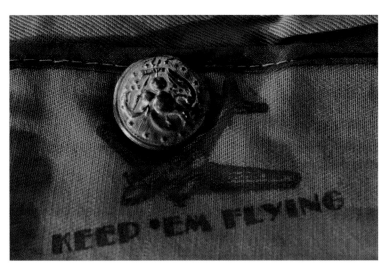

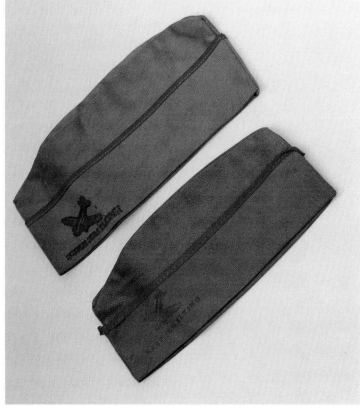

OS caps stamped with "Keep 'em Flying" were given away at bond and scrap drives to entice children to participate in the war effort.

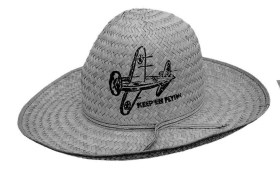

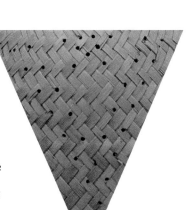

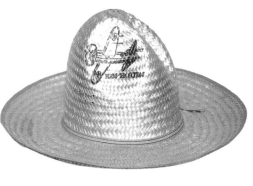

Straw hats stamped or stenciled with "Keep 'em Flying" were used as prizes at county fairs during the war. A victory "V" is punched out in tiny holes in the front of the straw hat from the left (center). *Courtesy Hank Brewer and Kathleen MacDonald Collection*

171

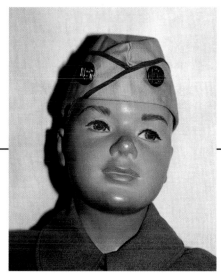

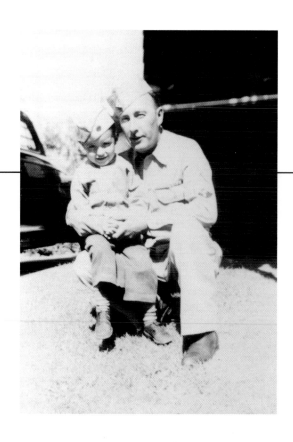

Fellow military-collectibles dealer Jim MacDonald was photographed in 1943 with his Uncle Archie, and also solo, showing off his store-bought visor and OS caps. Three-year-old Jim insisted his OS cap should have insignia on both sides, so his mother appeased the youngster by sewing a Michigan State Police button to the side of the cap. The cap (shown top left) is still owned by Jim and is a cherished item in his wife Kathleen's extensive children's military-uniform collection. *Courtesy Kathleen MacDonald Collection*

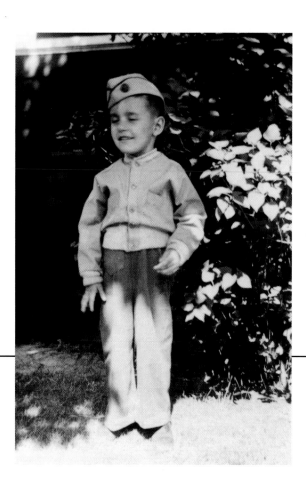

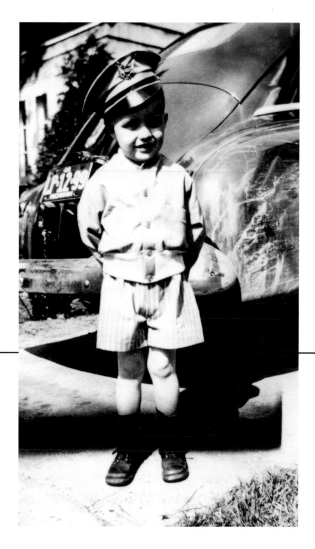

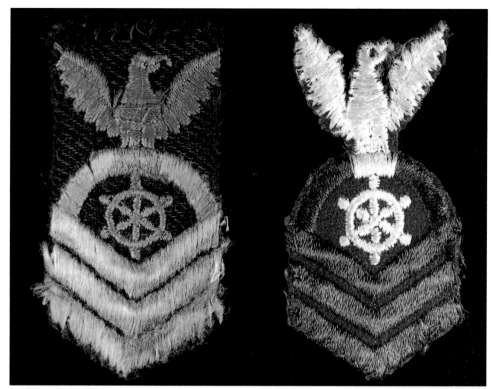

U.S. Navy chief quartermaster insignia probably removed from a child's uniform.

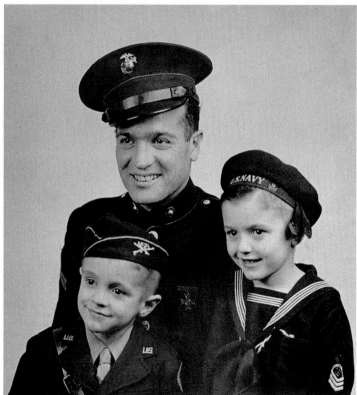

A photographic proof from a Steubenville, Ohio, photographic studio. The child on the right wears the same style insignia on his sleeve as the ones shown.

Right:
Walter Kanzler, military relics dealer *extraordinaire,* was only five years old when he posed in his handsome Navy whites in 1944. He later joined the U.S. Coast Guard and bravely defended the shores of his native New Jersey.

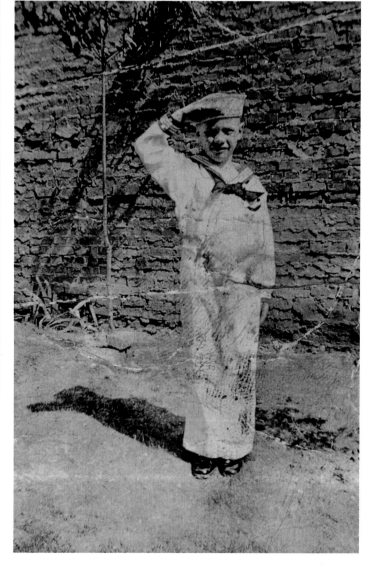

173

Post-World War II, Korea———

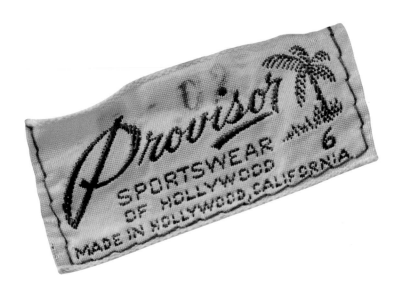

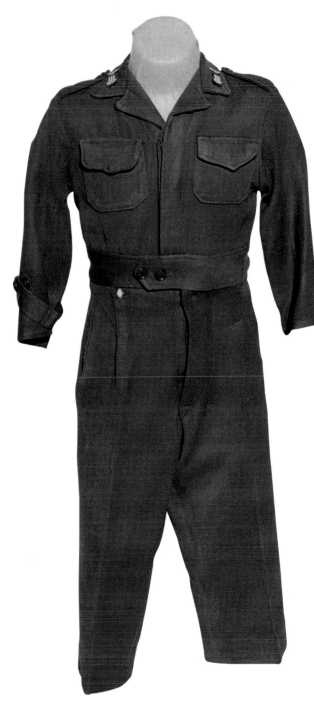

On July 22, 1954, David Eisenhower II receives a "parade drum" from Noble & Cooley Co. to celebrate the company's 100th anniversary. *Courtesy Noble & Cooley Co.*

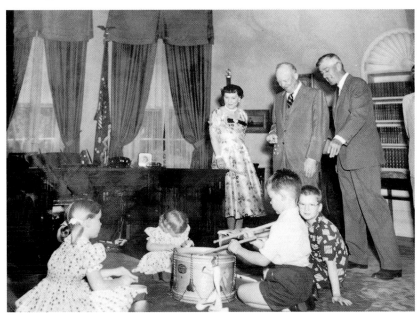

A post-war "Ike" tunic and trousers made by Provisor Sportswear of Hollywood, California.

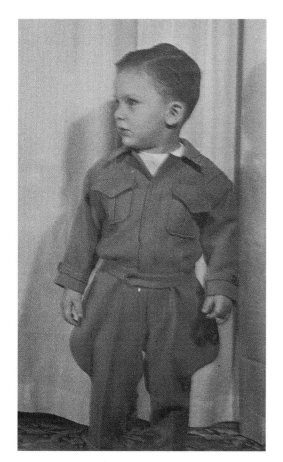

A photographic studio proof dated October 12, 1946. The riding-style trousers on this young man make the photo appear to be earlier than it really is.

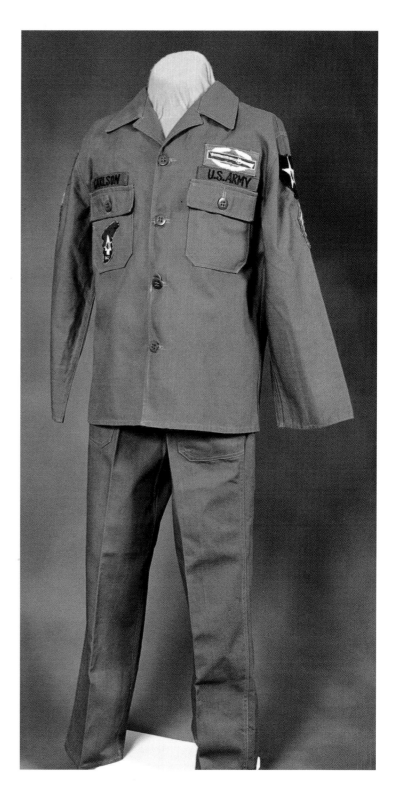

A mint example of a miniature uniform (right) replicated for the child of a serviceman stationed in Korea. The sleeve bears a 1st Division patch, and the pocket has an "Injun Scouts" patch and a DMZ patch, making the uniform very realistic and desirable. A pair of kid's aviator-style sunglasses and a Korean-era Matthew Ridgeway hat (right) whose manufacturer claims that it "lasts to the very end" complete the outfit.

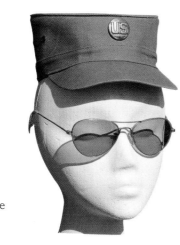

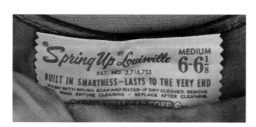

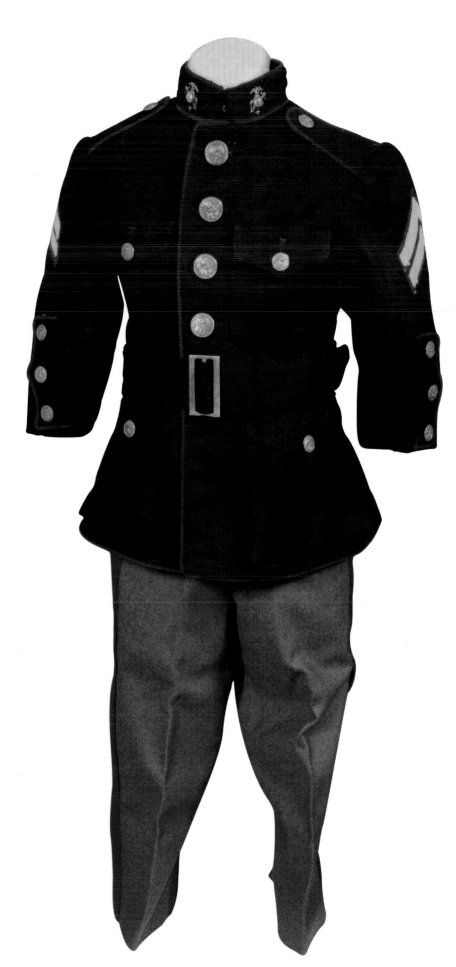

A beautifully detailed homemade wool U.S.M.C. dress uniform.

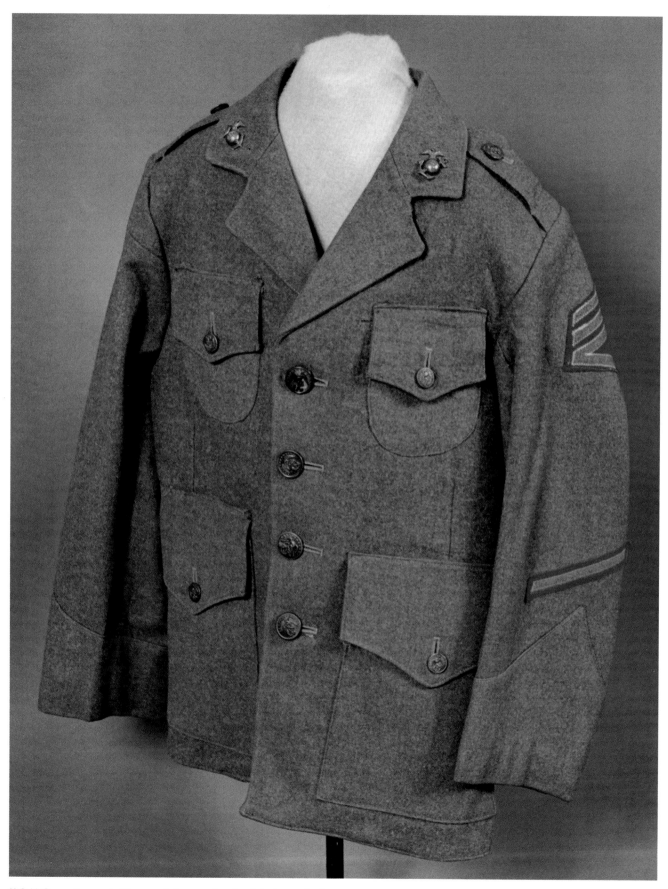

U.S.M.C. service coat. The regulation coats of enlisted men had belts. It is unknown if the one shown here ever had one.

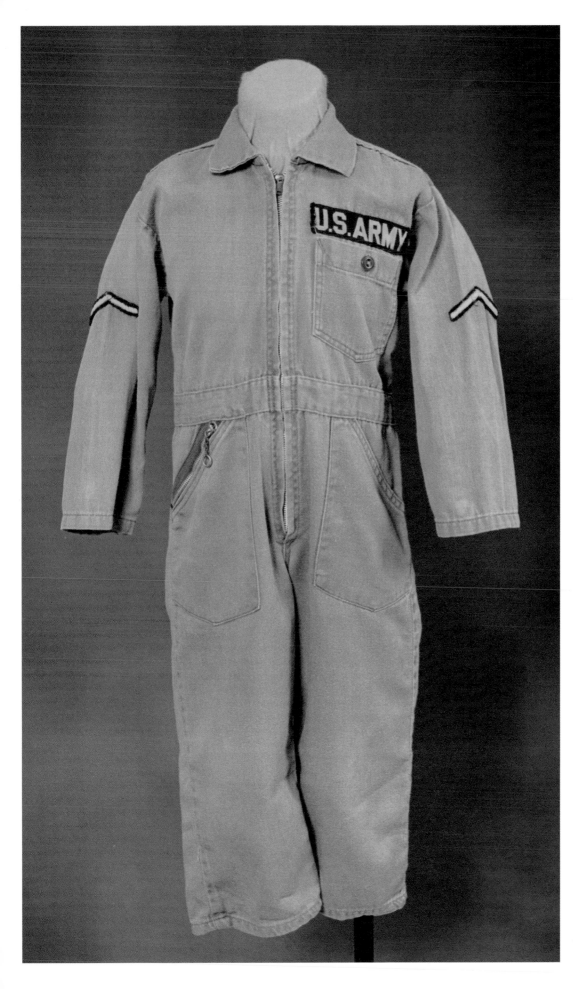

A one-piece herringbone twill coverall whose adult counterpart was used by the Army from WWII through the 1960s. This one most likely is of 1950s vintage.

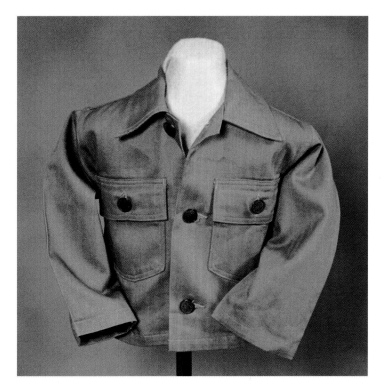

HBT Army shirt with standard army pattern "star of David" buttons typical of the World War II through Korea periods.

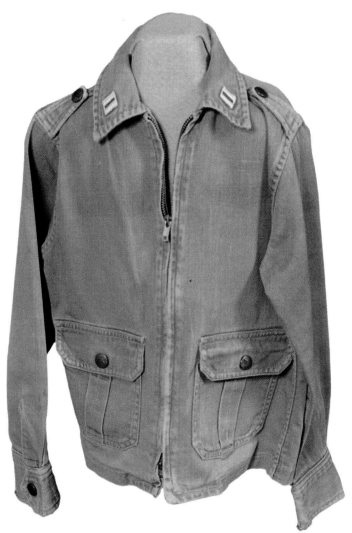

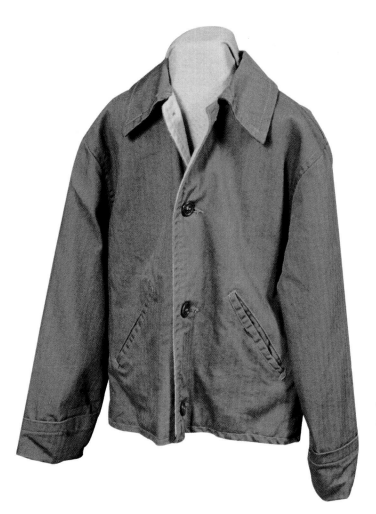

This civilian-style jacket has 1950s Air Force-style epaulets on the shoulders and captain's bars on the collar.

The two herringbone twill jackets above are military style (top) and civilian style (below).

179

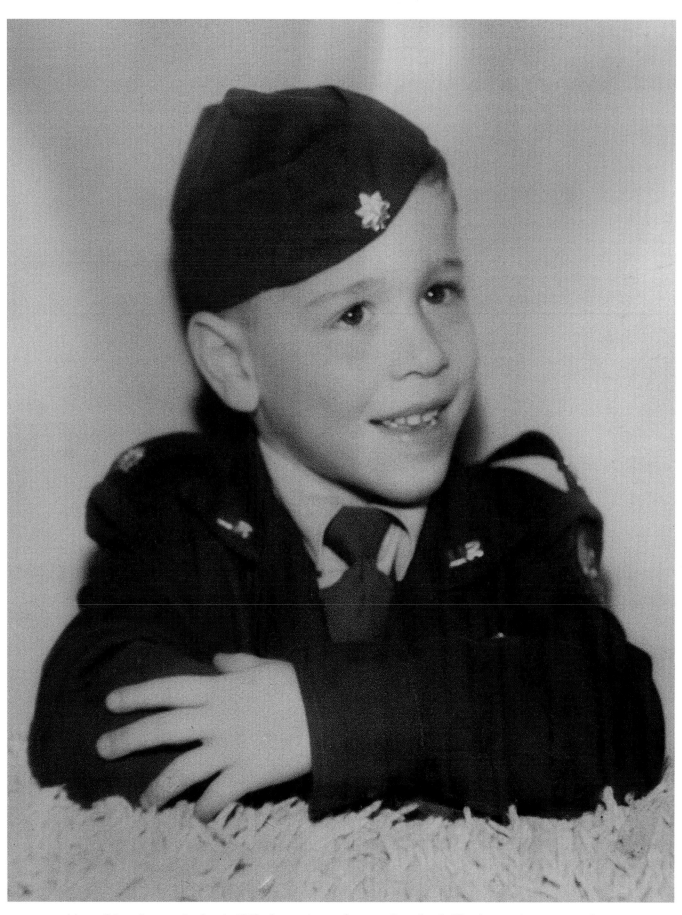

A beautiful studio portrait taken in 1952 of a young man from a military family. The Jr. major's insignia on the hat and epaulets have special meaning, since they belonged to different members of his immediate family. *Courtesy William Curtis*

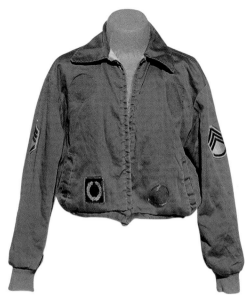

A lined tanker's-style jacket, which has had the many patches it once bore removed.

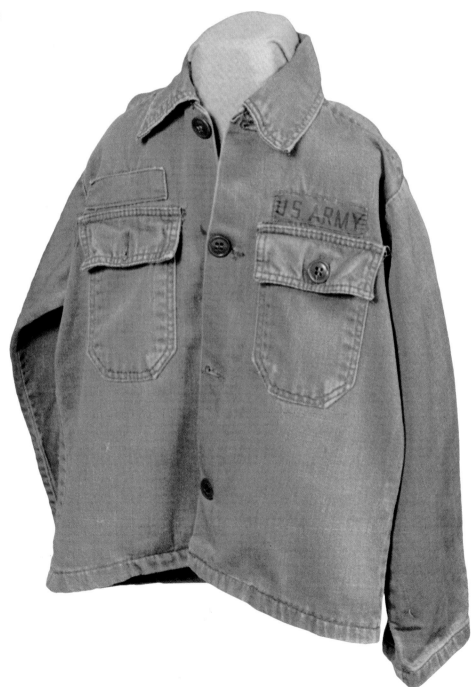

A sateen fatigue jacket style that was used by the U.S. Army from the late 1950s through the post-Vietnam era. This example would date after 1966, since it has dark name tags.

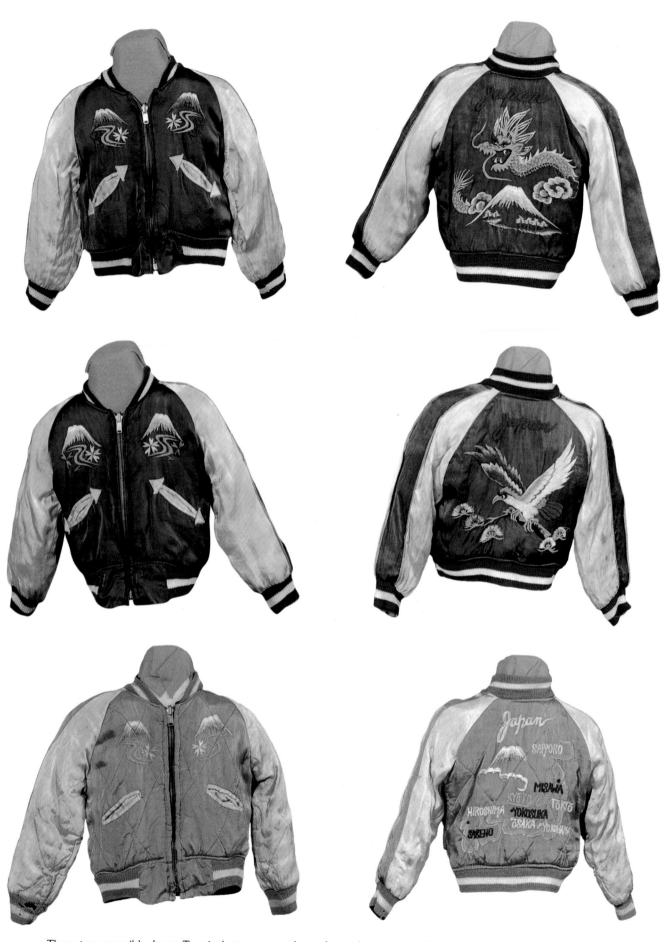

These two reversible Japan Tour jackets were sent home by an American serviceman to his twin boys in the early 1950s. Note the slight color variations in styling of embroidery and designs.

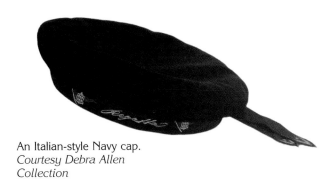

An Italian-style Navy cap.
Courtesy Debra Allen Collection

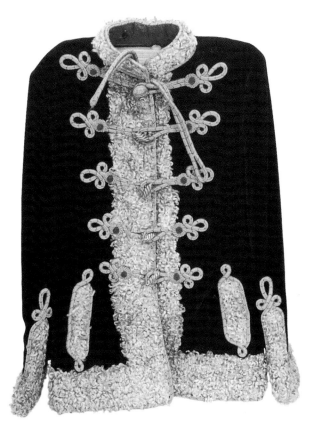

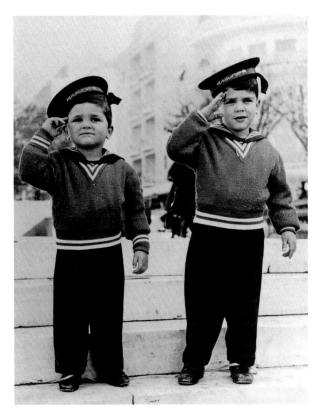

This tunic is 1950s English Hussar. It is sized to fit an eight- to ten-year-old child. This beautiful tunic is very fancy, produced from black velvet trimmed with genuine lamb's wool. The Hussar piping is gold with red highlights. The outfit most likely was made for the child of a wealthy officer. *Courtesy Marie DiMartini Whittmann Collection. Photo: Charles Jenkins, III*

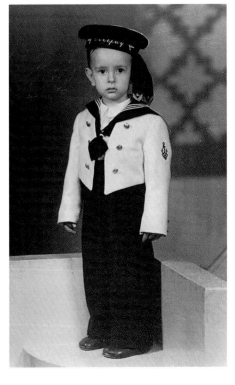

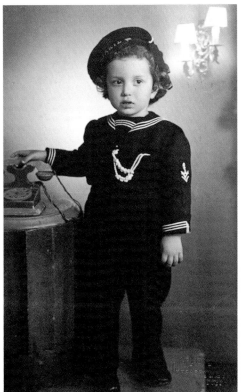

Above and right:
These four children in sailor suits were all photographed during the 1950s in Greece.

The Vietnam Era

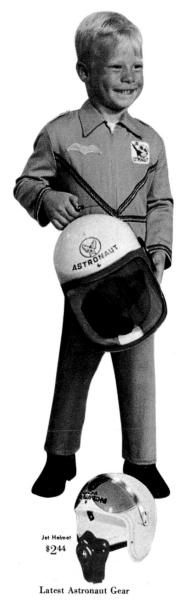

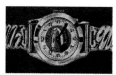

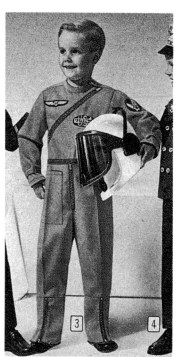

The space race was in full swing when Montgomery Ward offered its "Space Explorer Suit" in 1962. The "Steve Canyon Jet Helmet" made by the Ideal Toy Company in 1959 (inset) was another favorite for boys who wanted to enter the Jet Age and can still be readily found for collections. *Courtesy University of Wyoming American Heritage Center*

Jet Helmet
$2⁴⁴

Latest Astronaut Gear

1 **Ready For Count-Down!** Young space explorer's suit of sanforized cotton. Full zipper front; opens up or down; elastic back for better fit. Braid, embroid-ered astronaut insignias decorate front. Epaulets on shoulders. 2 large pockets. State size: Small, Medium, Large. See size chart, Page 320. *Astronaut Boots sold on opposite page.*
48 T 1740—Ship. wt. 12 oz.........**$3.94**

2 **Astronaut Helmet.** Sturdy forti-flex plastic with lift-up transparent face shield. Microphone mouthpiece, voice vibrator for "space" communication. Air Force emblem. Fits all head sizes.
48 T 1874—Ship. wt. 2 lbs..........**$3.33**

3 **Jet Helmet** of sturdy hi-impact plastic with lift-up sun visor and snap-on "oxygen mask." Fits all head sizes.
48 T 1737—Ship. wt. 1 lb...........**$2.44**

322 WARDS BACSK

Right and above right:
In 1961, Sears had an astronaut suit of its own. Both Sears and Montgomery Ward sold the essential astronaut helmet and boots separately (right). In 1966, Sears changed the silver-blue suit to a shiny, silvertone cotton twill (above) as the race to the moon heated up between the U.S. and Soviets. *Courtesy Sears Graphics*

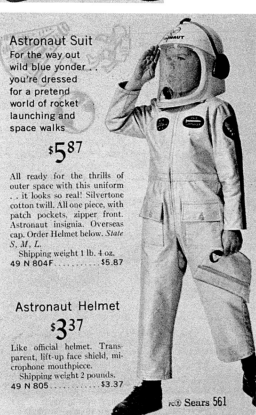

Astronaut Suit
For the way out wild blue yonder . . . you're dressed for a pretend world of rocket launching and space walks

$5⁸⁷

All ready for the thrills of outer space with this uniform . . it looks so real! Silvertone cotton twill. All one piece, with patch pockets, zipper front. Astronaut insignia. Overseas cap. Order Helmet below. *State S, M, L.*
Shipping weight 1 lb. 4 oz.
49 N 804F.........**$5.87**

Astronaut Helmet

$3³⁷

Like official helmet. Trans-parent, lift-up face shield, mi-crophone mouthpiece.
Shipping weight 2 pounds.
49 N 805...........**$3.37**

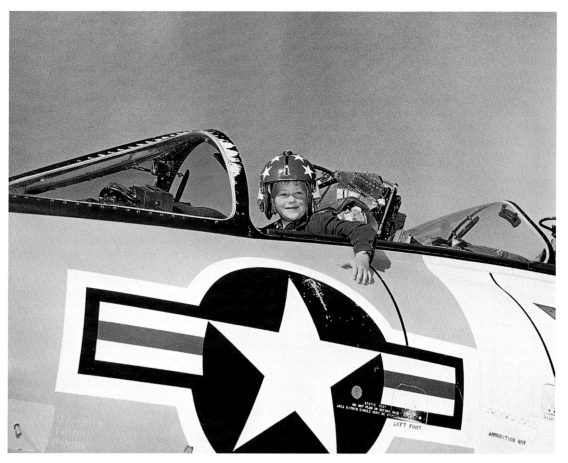

Rear Admiral Joseph Clifton hosted this young man's adventure of being photographed in a static fighter at the Naval Air Station at Corpus Christi, Texas, in February 1960. *Official U.S. Navy Photograph*

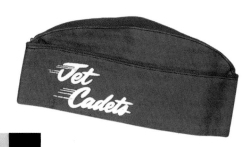

A great two-tone "Jet Cadets" OS cap, circa 1960s. *Courtesy Bob Chatt, Vintage Productions, Huntington Beach, California*

A complete store card of early 1960s U.S. military medals with plastic ribbons and no apparent way to affix them once they come out of their package. Note how the distinguished military man has a slight Asian appearance, given that they were "Made in Hong Kong."

185

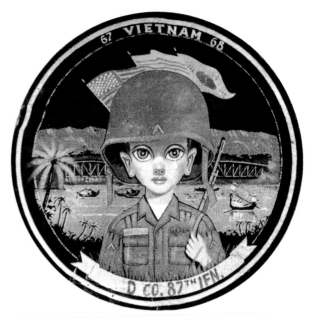

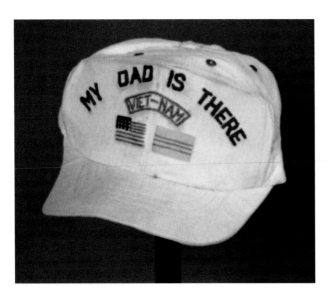

An in-country-made souvenir hat with direct-embroidered flags of the U.S. and South Vietnam.

Walter Keane was a popular artist from the 1960s who painted kids and animals with very large eyes. The local Vietnamese economy produced several would-be Keanes, mass-producing these childlike paintings of soldiers on velvet like this one shown. A soldier of any ethnic background could be purchased and his name, unit, and rank quickly penned or painted in to complete the souvenir.

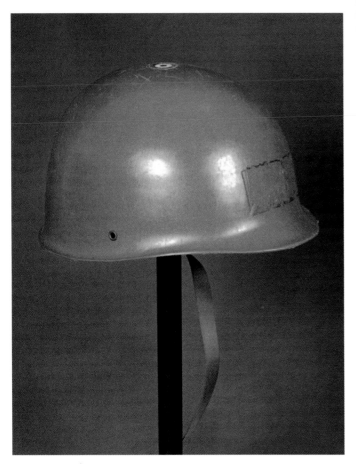

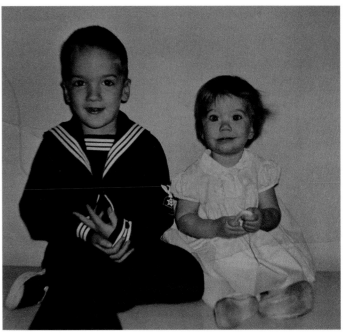

The photo of these two children is in a tiny wallet-size format, possibly to be sent to a family member serving overseas during the 1960s.

Opposite page:
Major Darel D. Leetun was an F105D Thunderchief pilot who had this flight suit made and sent home from Vietnam for his young daughter. He was assigned a combat mission over North Vietnam on September 17, 1966. When Leetun was over Lang Son Province about halfway between the cities of Kep and Loc Binh, the aircraft was shot down. As of the printing of this book, his official status remains MIA by the United States Government.

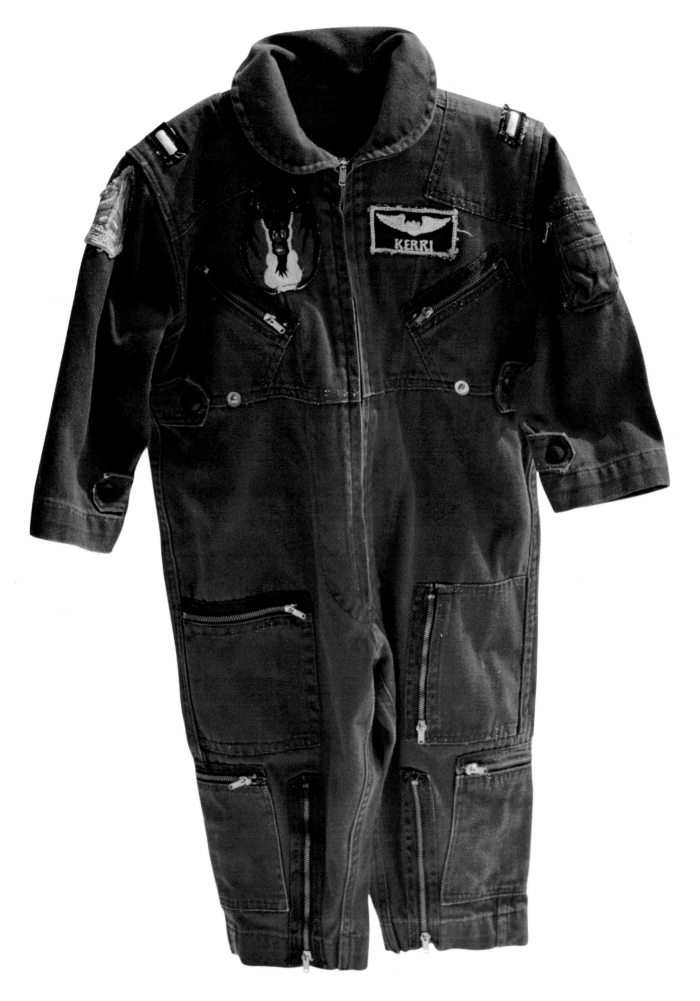

187

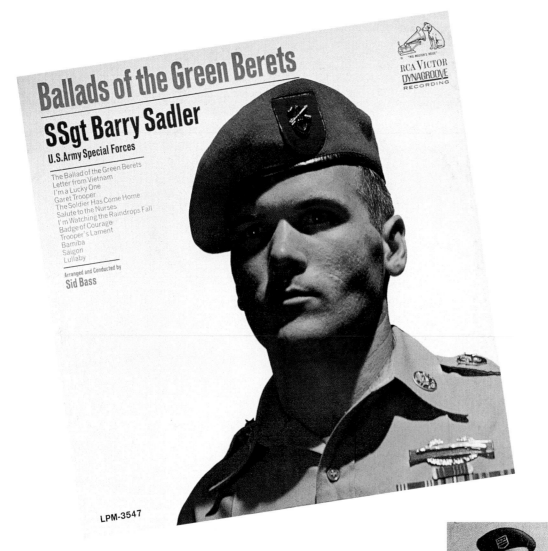

Ballads of the Green Berets

SSgt Barry Sadler
U.S. Army Special Forces

The Ballad of the Green Berets
Letter from Vietnam
I'm a Lucky One
Garet Trooper
The Soldier Has Come Home
Salute to the Nurses
I'm Watching the Raindrops Fall
Badge of Courage
Trooper's Lament
Bamiba
Saigon
Lullaby

Arranged and Conducted by
Sid Bass

LPM-3547

The success of Barry Saddler's "The Ballad of the Green Berets" may have been what inspired costume companies to produce Green Beret playsuits in time for the Christmas catalogs in 1966, the same year the album debuted. *Courtesy Sears Graphics*

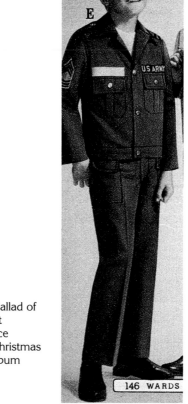

146 WARDS

Outfit	Hat
$4.94	$1.00

Outfit Plus Hat
$5.66

E He'll be in the famous Green Berets with this U. S. Army Special Forces Outfit. 100% cotton twill "Ike" jacket, epaulet shoulders. Name tape. Rank insignias. Olive. Machine wash, medium. Sizes: 4, 6, 8, 10, 12. State size.
Z 33 T 2661 Outfit Wt. 1 lb...$4.94

Green Beret. Wool Felt. Wt. 4 oz. 33 T 1610-1 size fits all.....$1.00
Z 33 T 2666—Outfit and Hat. Wt. 1 lb. 4 oz. State size of outfit...$5.66

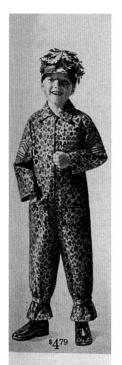

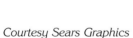

Ranger. 1-pc. cotton twill camouflage suit, full zipper. Insignia. Plastic helmet. *State size* S, M, L. Shipping wt. 1 lb. 8 oz.
49 N 802F $4.79

122 SEARS PCBL

Courtesy Sears Graphics

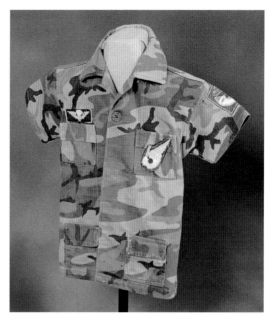

Child's ARVN Ranger BDQ (Biet Dong Quan) shirt and trousers. The shirt has jump-status wing and Viet-Airborne Division patches.

Courtesy Sears Graphics

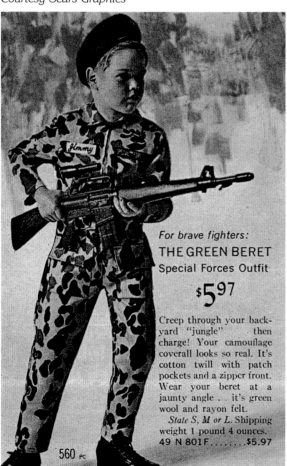

For brave fighters:
THE GREEN BERET
Special Forces Outfit

$5.97

Creep through your backyard "jungle" then charge! Your camouflage coverall looks so real. It's cotton twill with patch pockets and a zipper front. Wear your beret at a jaunty angle . . . it's green wool and rayon felt.
State S, M or L. Shipping weight 1 pound 4 ounces.
49 N 801F $5.97

560 PC

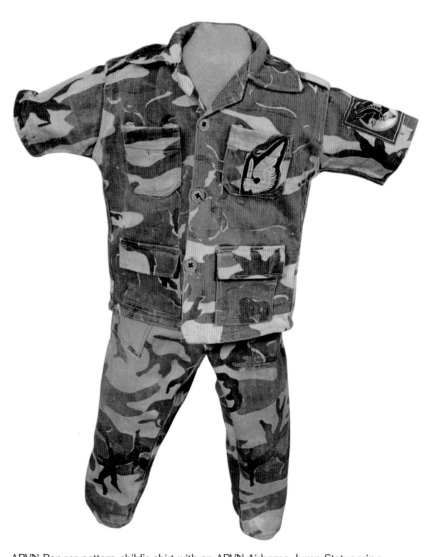

ARVN Ranger-pattern child's shirt with an ARVN Airborne Jump Status wing.

189

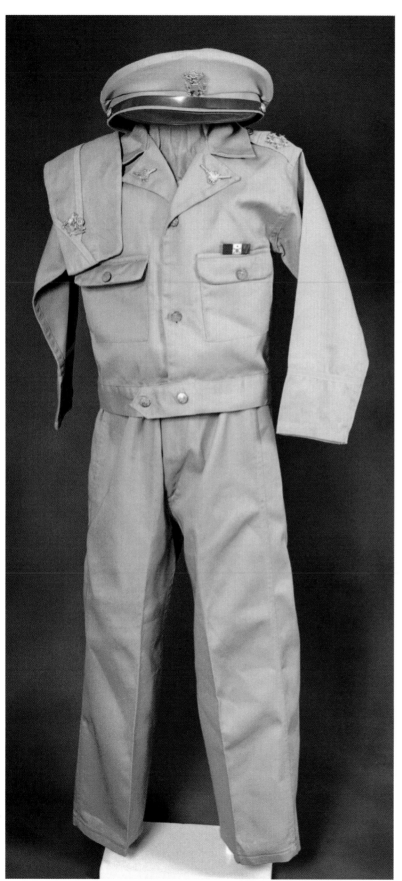

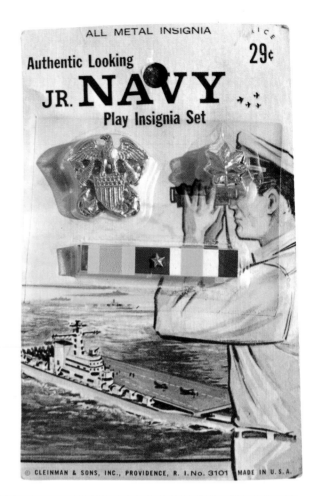

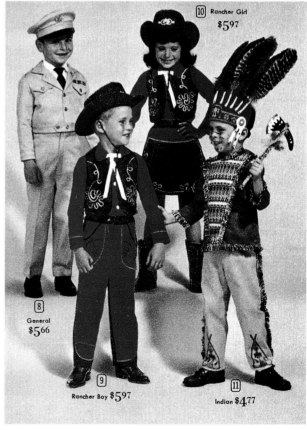

Five-star general's uniform like the one shown right is from the
Montgomery Ward Catalog, circa 1961.

Courtesy University of Wyoming American Heritage Center

190

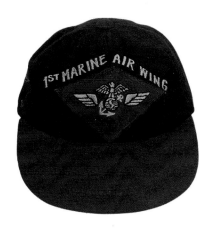

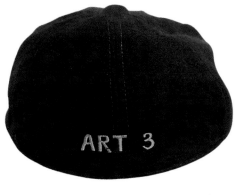

This child's Vietnam-era 1st Marine Air Wing Division wool ball cap was made in Japan. The "call sign" of the owner's dad is embroidered on the reverse. *Courtesy Bob Chatt, Vintage Productions, Huntington Beach, California*

Jumpsuit with a 3rd Marine Air Wing patch on the breast and a kid-size "Boonie"-style hat. *Courtesy Debra Allan Collection*

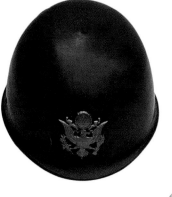

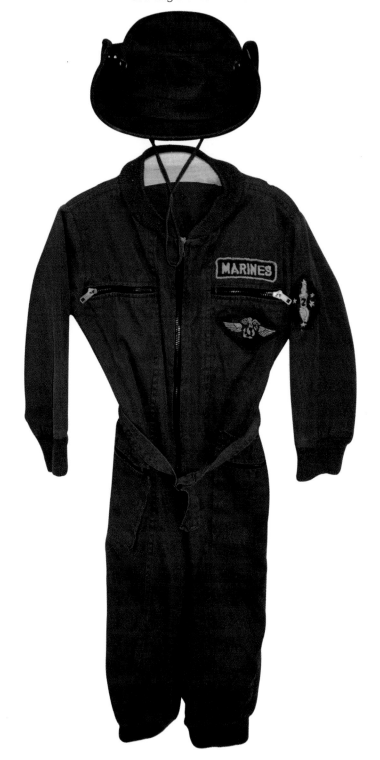

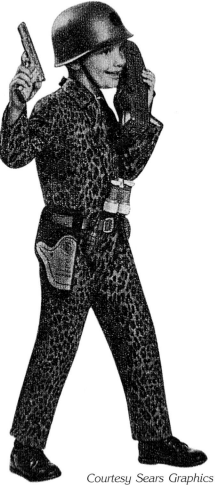

Courtesy Sears Graphics

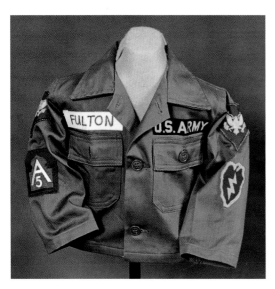

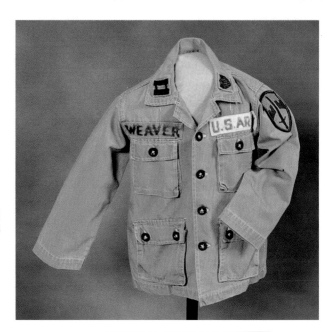

Left:
OG-107 sateen jacket from the early 1960s.

Right:
A very small kid's Army-style shirt with appliqued insignia and a post-1968 subdued MACV Adjutant General's Corps patch on the shoulder.

Allie Tabor shows off her Vietnam-style outfit and gear at the TMCA Military Collectibles Show in Nashville, Tennessee, where her dad buys and sells military relics with hundreds of others on Thanksgiving and Easter weekends at the National Guard Armory.

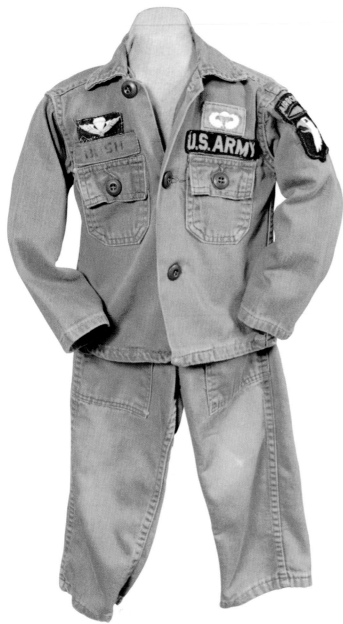

An in-country-made shirt and trousers with a pre-1968 Viet Jump Wing and 101st Airborne Division on the sleeve.

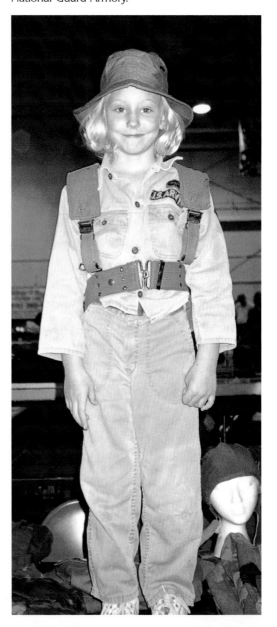

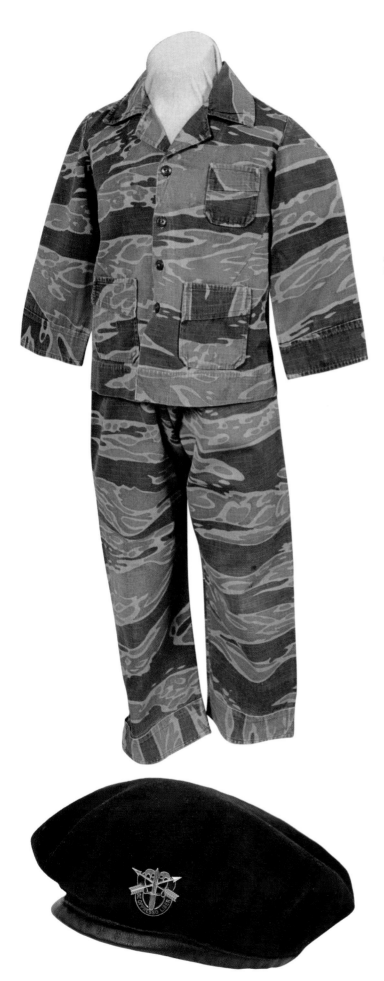

A late- to post-Vietnam American tiger-stripe-pattern shirt and pants.

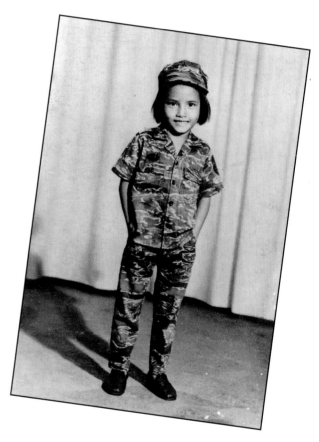

The pattern for the coarse lightweight tiger-stripe camo this Vietnamese girl is wearing dates in the early 1970s. Hundreds of photos like this from Saigon photo studios made their way to America when military relics dealers made post-war buying trips to Southeast Asia in the 1980s.

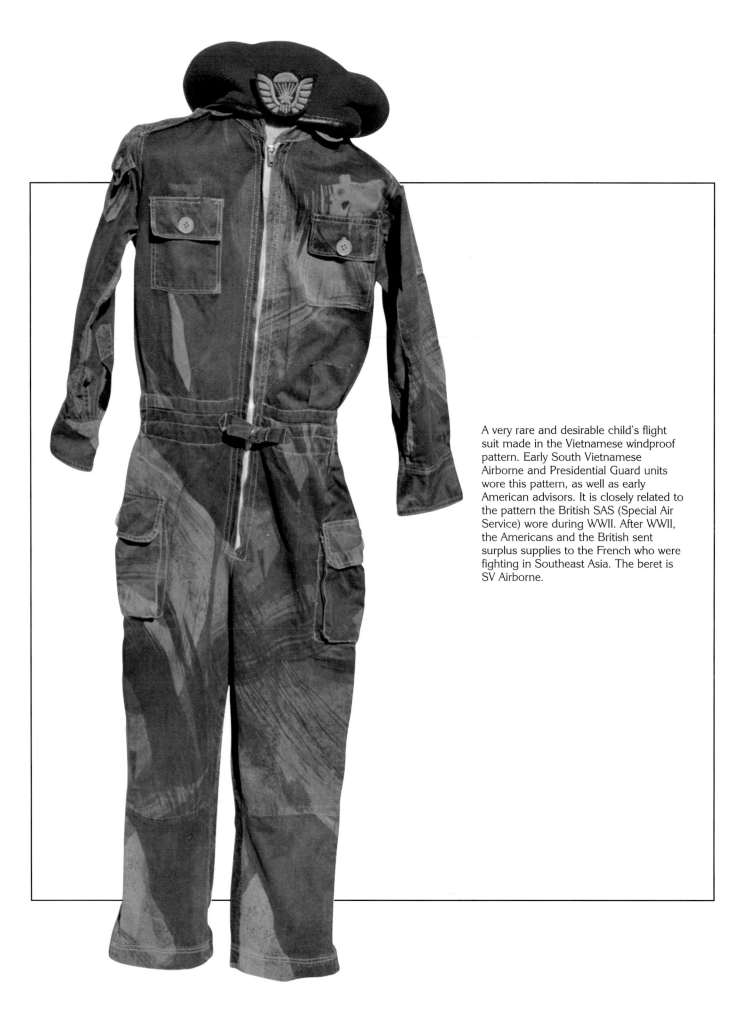

A very rare and desirable child's flight suit made in the Vietnamese windproof pattern. Early South Vietnamese Airborne and Presidential Guard units wore this pattern, as well as early American advisors. It is closely related to the pattern the British SAS (Special Air Service) wore during WWII. After WWII, the Americans and the British sent surplus supplies to the French who were fighting in Southeast Asia. The beret is SV Airborne.

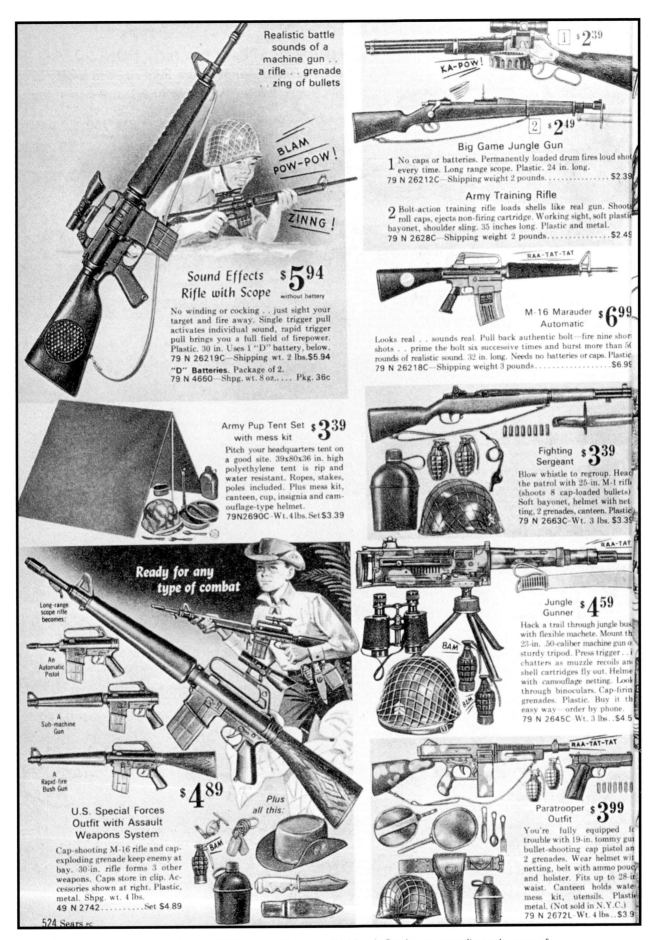

Realistic battle sounds of a machine gun .. a rifle .. grenade .. zing of bullets

BLAM POW-POW!

ZINNG!

KA-POW!

Big Game Jungle Gun

1 $2³⁹ No caps or batteries. Permanently loaded drum fires loud shot every time. Long range scope. Plastic. 24 in. long.
79 N 26212C—Shipping weight 2 pounds.............$2.39

Army Training Rifle

2 $2⁴⁹ Bolt-action training rifle loads shells like real gun. Shoots roll caps, ejects non-firing cartridge. Working sight, soft plastic bayonet, shoulder sling. 35 inches long. Plastic and metal.
79 N 2628C—Shipping weight 2 pounds.............$2.49

Sound Effects Rifle with Scope $5⁹⁴ without battery

No winding or cocking .. just sight your target and fire away. Single trigger pull activates individual sound, rapid trigger pull brings you a full field of firepower. Plastic. 30 in. Uses 1 "D" battery, below.
79 N 26219C—Shipping wt. 2 lbs.$5.94
"D" Batteries. Package of 2.
79 N 4660—Shpg. wt. 8 oz..... Pkg. 36c

RAA-TAT-TAT

M-16 Marauder Automatic $6⁹⁹

Looks real .. sounds real. Pull back authentic bolt—fire nine short shots .. prime the bolt six successive times and burst more than 50 rounds of realistic sound. 32 in. long. Needs no batteries or caps. Plastic
79 N 26218C—Shipping weight 3 pounds...............$6.99

Army Pup Tent Set $3³⁹ with mess kit

Pitch your headquarters tent on a good site. 39x80x36 in. high polyethylene tent is rip and water resistant. Ropes, stakes, poles included. Plus mess kit, canteen, cup, insignia and camouflage-type helmet.
79N2690C—Wt.4 lbs.Set $3.39

Fighting Sergeant $3³⁹

Blow whistle to regroup. Head the patrol with 25-in. M-1 rifle (shoots 8 cap-loaded bullets) Soft bayonet, helmet with netting, 2 grenades, canteen. Plastic.
79 N 2663C-Wt. 3 lbs. $3.39

Ready for any type of combat

Long-range scope rifle becomes:

An Automatic Pistol

A Sub-machine Gun

A Rapid-fire Bush Gun

BAM

$4⁸⁹

Plus all this:

U.S. Special Forces Outfit with Assault Weapons System

Cap-shooting M-16 rifle and cap-exploding grenade keep enemy at bay. 30-in. rifle forms 3 other weapons. Caps store in clip. Accessories shown at right. Plastic, metal. Shpg. wt. 4 lbs.
49 N 2742..........Set $4.89

RAA-TAT

Jungle Gunner $4⁵⁹

Hack a trail through jungle bush with flexible machete. Mount the 23-in. .50-caliber machine gun on sturdy tripod. Press trigger .. it chatters as muzzle recoils and shell cartridges fly out. Helmet with camouflage netting. Look through binoculars. Cap-firing grenades. Plastic. Buy it the easy way—order by phone.
79 N 2645C-Wt. 3 lbs.-$4.59

BAM

RAA-TAT-TAT

Paratrooper Outfit $3⁹⁹

You're fully equipped for trouble with 19-in. tommy gun, bullet-shooting cap pistol and 2 grenades. Wear helmet with netting, belt with ammo pouch and holster. Fits up to 28-in. waist. Canteen holds water, mess kit, utensils. Plastic, metal. (Not sold in N.Y.C.)
79 N 2672L-Wt. 4 lbs ..$3.99

Most of the toys appearing on this mid-1960s Sears Christmas Wishbook Catalog page replicate the type of equipment American servicemen were using at the time. Note that a Vietnam-style "Boonie" hat is included in the Special Forces Assault Weapons System (lower left). *Courtesy Sears Graphics*

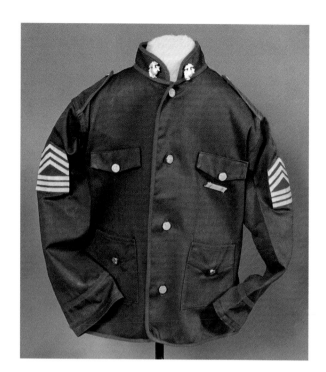

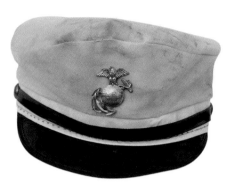

From the early to late 1960s, toy manufacturers offered a variety of U.S.M.C. dress blues. Over the years the quality gradually declined.

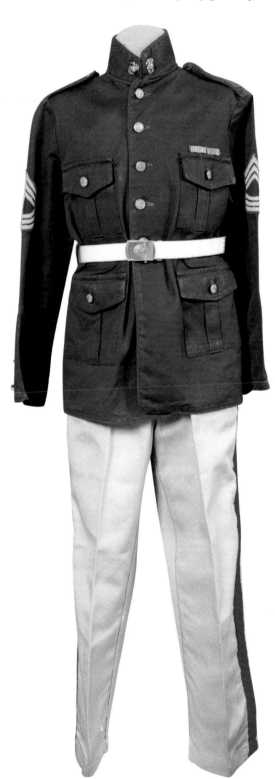

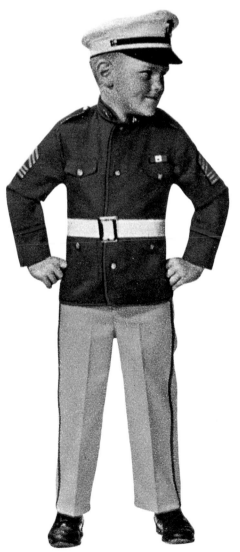

Courtesy University of Wyoming American Heritage Center

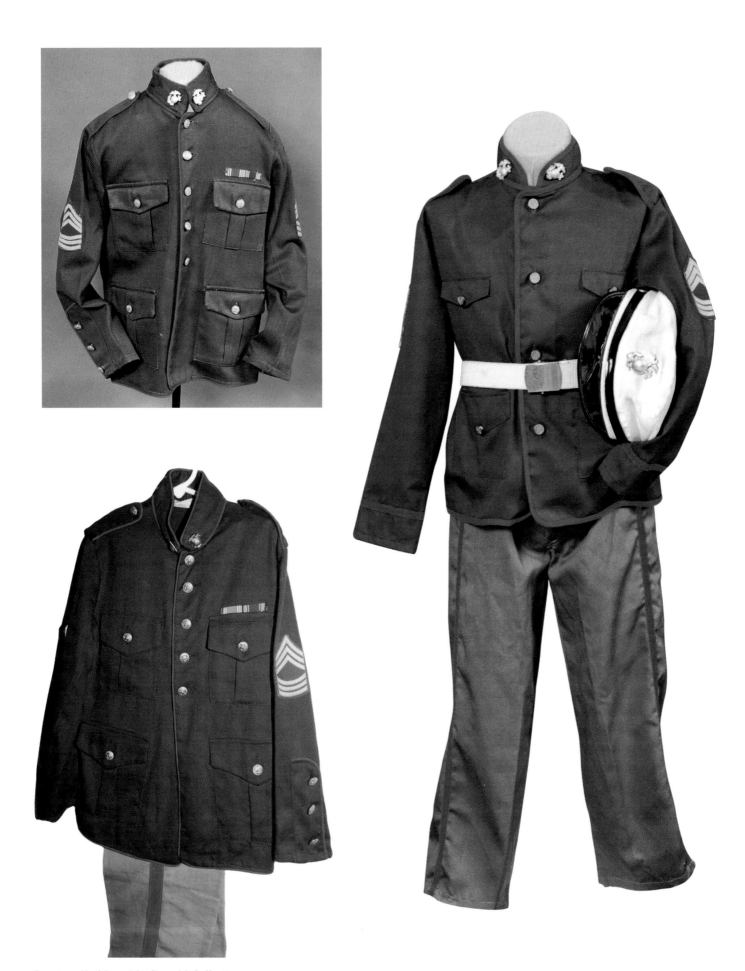

Courtesy Kathleen MacDonald Collection

197

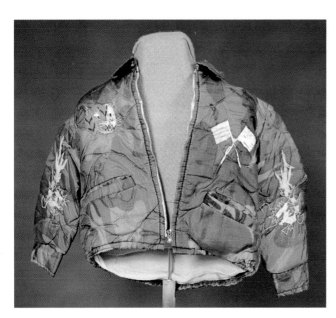
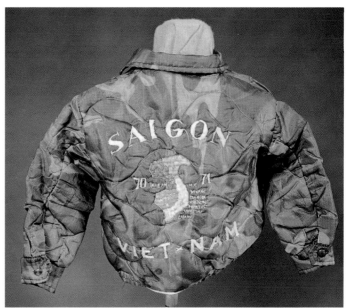

A quilted camo tour jacket. These jackets were purchased by servicemen in the shops of Saigon in sizes for themselves as well as their children.

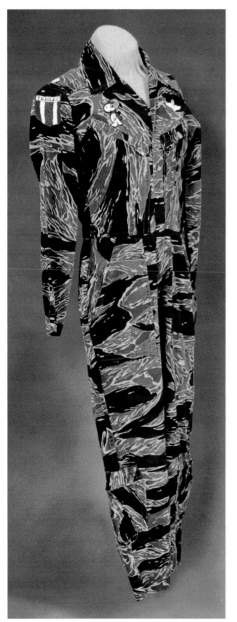
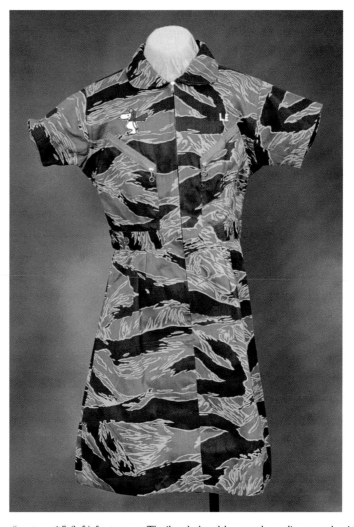

A Thai-tiger "party suit" (left) features a Thailand shoulder patch, a direct-embroidered senior pilot wing, and Snoopy dressed as his WWI Flying Ace alter ego. The seldom seen Thai-tiger dress features a more highly stylized version of the Snoopy character and the "LE" (Asian name) over the breast pockets. The Peanuts characters, especially Snoopy, were popular subjects for patches designed by military personnel during the Vietnam era, much like Disney and Tex Avery characters were popular during WWII. (Peanuts comic strip characters are a copyright of United Feature Syndicate, Inc.)

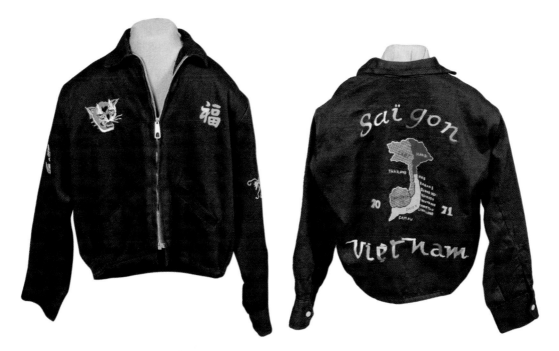

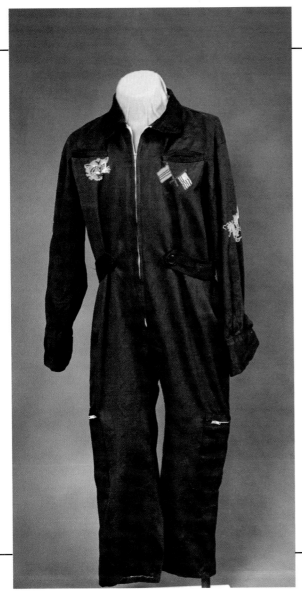

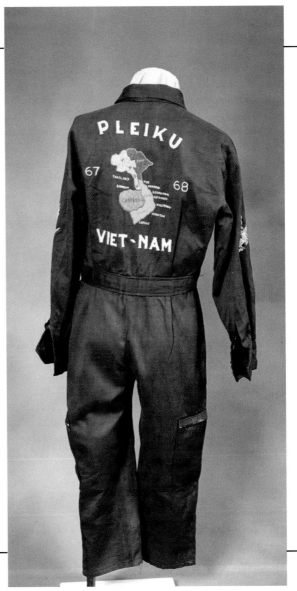

"Party jackets" and suits such as these are replicas of adult-size suits sent home to children. American service personnel (especially pilots) often wore these types of jackets and suits while (partying) off-duty.

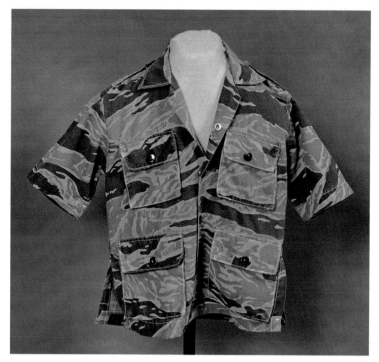

Philippines-pattern tiger stripe.

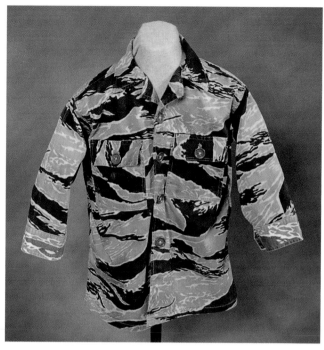

An interesting Viet-Marine tiger-stripe shirt whose cuffs are in a different pattern from the rest of the shirt.

Kids in Camo

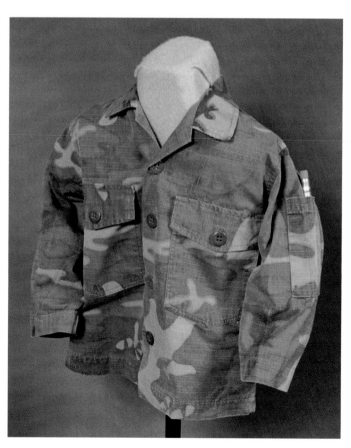

Post-1969 ARVN (Army Republic of Vietnam) ERDL pattern—experimental.

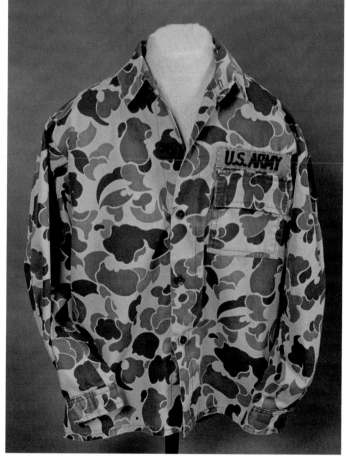

A civilian camouflage pattern.

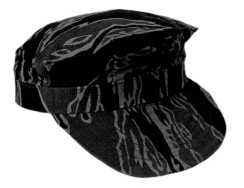
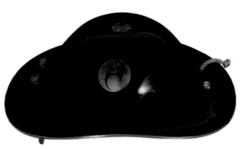
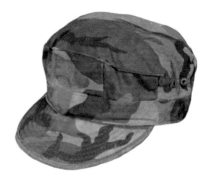

The hats on the ends are in-country made. The one on the right has had a small amount of dirt from Vietnam sewn into a pouch at the back of the brim. A circa 1970s child-size lacquered Japanese samurai helmet (center).

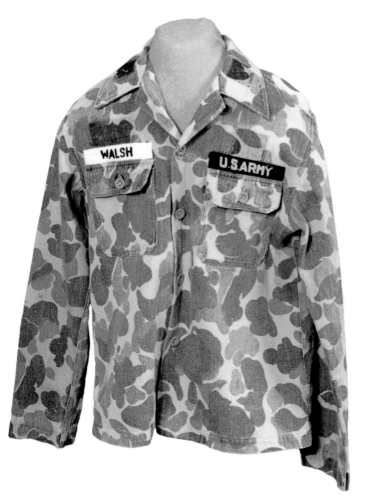

An early (1963 to 1965) in-country-made "duck"-pattern shirt.

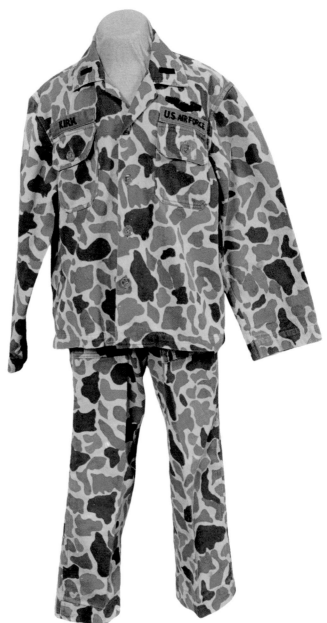

Another duck pattern used from 1968 to 1971. The name strip is the Air Force pilot subdued type. This style could be found and purchased in any tailor shop in Asia. The shirt and pants are sized to fit a child of about six to eight years old.

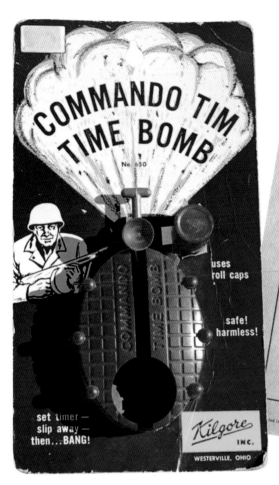

COMMANDO TIM TIME BOMB

No. 650

...uses roll caps

...safe! harmless!

set timer —
slip away —
then...BANG!

Kilgore INC.
WESTERVILLE, OHIO

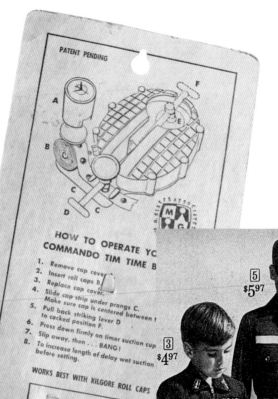

PATENT PENDING

HOW TO OPERATE YOUR
COMMANDO TIM TIME BOMB

1. Remove cap cover.
2. Insert roll caps B.
3. Replace cap cover.
4. Slide cap strip under prongs C.
   Make sure cap is centered between t
5. Pull back striking lever D
   to cocked position F.
6. Press down firmly on timer suction cup
7. Slip away, then . . . BANG!
8. To increase length of delay wet suction
   before setting.

WORKS BEST WITH KILGORE ROLL CAPS

Kilgore INC.
WESTERVILLE, OHIO

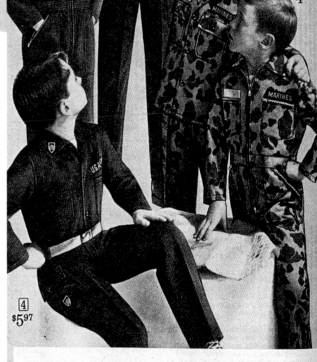

ATTEN . . SHUN! Your
boy will have hours of
fun with these rugged,
life-like Army
and Marine
play uniforms

3 — $4.97
5 — $5.97
6 — $5.97
7 — $4.97
4 — $5.97

Army style . . cotton corduroy. Heavyweight . . with double knees for extra protection. Authentic olive-drab color. Sanforized®. Machine washable, medium temperature.

3 Coverall Jumpsuit.
State size 4, 6, 8, 10 or 12.
40 N 65671F—Shipping weight 1 lb....$4.97

4 2-piece Fatigue Suit . . jacket, pants.
State size 4, 6, 8, 10 or 12.
40 N 65670F—Shpg. wt. 1 lb. 6 oz....$5.97

Army style . . cotton sateen. Olive drab color. Sanforized . . maximum fabric shrinkage 1%. Machine washable, medium temperature.

5 3-piece Fatigue Suit . . includes jacket, pants and cap.
State size 4, 6, 8, 10 or 12.
40 N 65640F—Shpg. wt. 1 lb. 6 oz....$5.97

Marine style . . cotton twill. Authentic camouflage coloring will give boys hours of fun . . hides them from "enemy". . blends in with natural surroundings. Sanforized . . maximum fabric shrinkage 1%. Machine wash, medium.

6 3-piece Jungle Outfit . . includes jacket, pants and cap.
State size 4, 6, 8, 10 or 12.
40 N 65650F—Shpg. wt. 1 lb. 6 oz....$5.97

7 Coverall Jumpsuit . . gives boy fullest protection from soil.
State size 4, 6, 8, 10 or 12.
40 N 65651F—Shipping weight 1 lb....$4.97

Marine-style Cap. Sizes S(6¼-6⅜); M(6½-6⅝); L(6¾-6⅞). See boys' size chart, Fall Catalog, page 892.
State size S, M or L.
40 N 65658F—Shipping weight 2 oz....97c

This Cold War toy was offered for the kids of the "Duck 'n' Cover" generation.

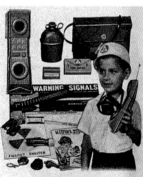

Civilian Defense Set $3.99

Send "messages" over the plastic walkie talkie set . . tack up signs and set up your own shelter. Dress up in your white helmet, belt and arm band like a regular civilian defense worker. Set also includes bag with emergency rations, play gas mask respirator, play radiation tester, canteen, flashlight, whistle, first aid manual and more.
49 N 1793—Shpg. wt. 2 lbs....$3.99

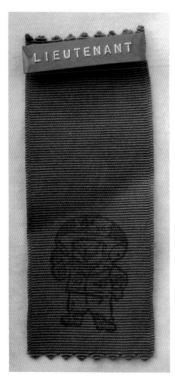

LIEUTENANT

A homemade badge for a little jet pilot. *Courtesy Bob Chatt, Vintage Productions, Huntington Beach, California*

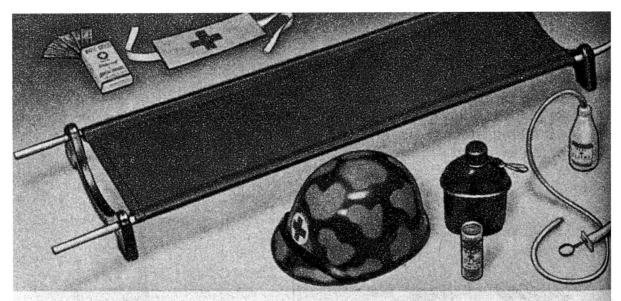

Rescue is on the way with this Corpsman Set $7⁷⁷

Be a front-lines medic with this 8-pc. medical corpsman outfit. You can actually carry the "wounded". Set 5-foot stretcher down on its rigid plastic legs. Give battlefield "casualty" water from canteen, hypo "shot," "plasma" transfusion—even pills that taste like candy. Bandage "wounds" and lift him onto the sturdy cotton-and-steel stretcher. Wear the adjustable plastic camouflaged helmet and medic armband. All in military colors.

79 N 1863C—Shipping weight 9 pounds....................................$7.77

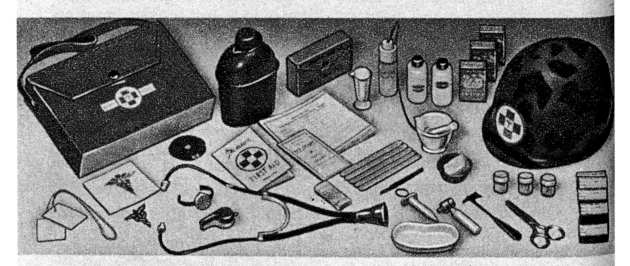

60-piece Combat Medical Kit $3⁹⁹

Just like the army medics on TV . . a modern-day outfit complete with all basic requirements used by the army medics. Plastic helmet, plastic canteen, 2 "dog tags" with chain, first aid kit, sound stethoscope, hypo needle, blood plasma bottle, emblem pin and whistle, plus 50 medical items for "Battlefield" care.

49 N 1699—Shipping weight 2 pounds....................................$3.99

Signs of the times. Though these toys may seem a little disturbing now, these two sets merely replicated the types of things families watched on the evening news and weekly television programs during the conflict in Vietnam. The kit (lower) even states: "Just like the Army medics on TV." *Courtesy Sears Graphics*

A great Indian Wars play set offered by Sears in 1967, the same year American families were watching Ken Berry head the command of "bumbling Cavalrymen and inept Indians" on ABC's F-Troop. *Courtesy Sears Graphics*

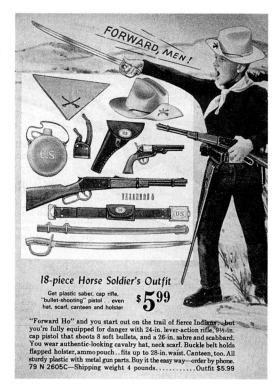

18-piece Horse Soldier's Outfit

Get plastic saber, cap rifle, "bullet-shooting" pistol .. even hat, scarf, canteen and holster

$5.99

"Forward Ho" and you start out on the trail of fierce Indians . . but you're fully equipped for danger with 24-in. lever-action rifle, 9½-in. cap pistol that shoots 8 soft bullets, and a 26-in. sabre and scabbard. You wear authentic-looking cavalry hat, neck scarf. Buckle belt holds flapped holster, ammo pouch . . fits up to 28-in. waist. Canteen, too. All sturdy plastic with metal gun parts. Buy it the easy way—order by phone.
79 N 2605C—Shipping weight 4 pounds............Outfit $5.99

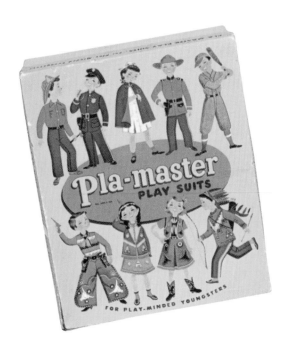

Several companies that manufactured children's costumes produced versions of the Federal and Confederate Army uniforms during the Civil War Centennial, celebrated from 1961 to1965. The higher quality cotton-flannel Confederate uniform (below) was made by Nattyboys Gallant Grey, while the blue cotton-twill Union uniform (top, opposite page) was offered by Pla-Master and is the same uniform shown in the Sears Catalog page (below, opposite page)

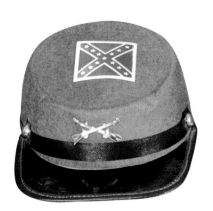

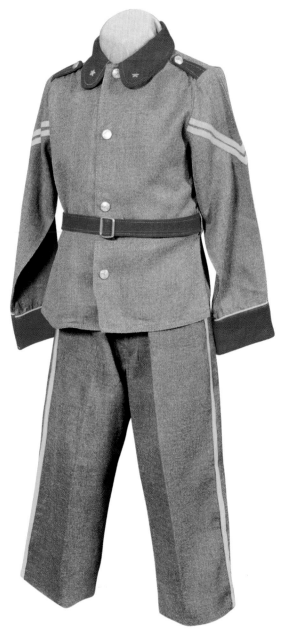

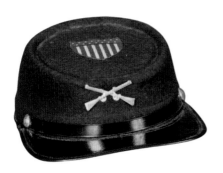

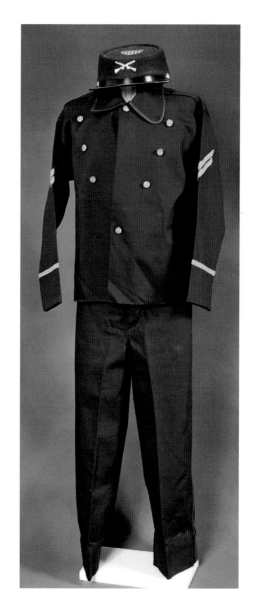

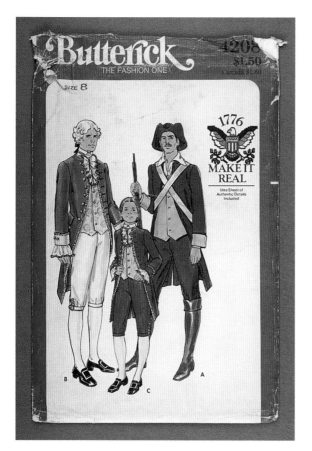

Butterick Patterns offers an opportunity for another generation of Americans to celebrate the next century mark of the birth of our nation in true Revolutionary style.

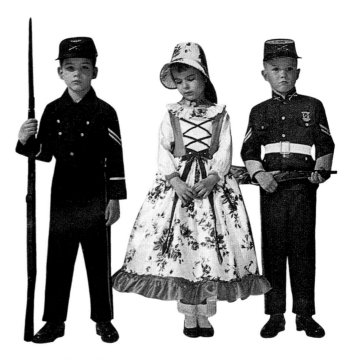

Courtesy Sears Graphics

205

Glossary

AEF. Australian Expeditionary Forces. Australian Expeditionary Forces I and II were the Army of Australia during World War I and World War II.

ambrotype. Negative image produced on glass and viewed as a positive by inclusion of a black background.

ARVN. Army Republic of Vietnam.

AVG. American Volunteer Group. The pilots and crews who volunteered services to China to fight against the Japanese prior to American involvement in World War II.

backmark. A trademark used by photographers on CDV images to identify their studio. Later many photographers switched the mark to the front where it could be seen along with the image. On buttons, the backmark refers to the manufacturer's name and/or trademark stamped into the back of a button.

blockade runner. Opportunist merchants and patriots who bring in supplies through a military blockade to aid the allied cause.

boatswain. Directs and supervises men in marlinespike and deck and boat seamanship; he paints, maintains the ship, and looks after the rigging, deck equipment, and boats.

bullion. The gold thread overlay used to make insignia. Favored for military regalia.

bummer (kepi). Typical enlisted forage cap named because of the amount of fabric needed to make the cap and the slope of the peak that falls forward.

cabinet card. Style of photography denoted by an image glued to heavy cardstock measuring 4-1/2 inches by 6-1/2 inches.

CBI. China, Burma, India. Refers to the theater of operation during World War II and patch worn by servicemen assigned to the theater.

CDV. *Carte de viste.* An albumen print mounted on a 2-1/4 inch x 4-1/4 inch piece of lightweight cardboard. CDV photography was popular from the 1850s to the 1860s.

chasseur. French for heavy cavalry.

chechia. A turban-wrapped fez.

coxswain. A sailor assigned to steer a boat. He is also in charge of the boat's crew.

cuirassier. German for heavy cavalry.

degan. German for sword.

Dewey suit. A suit made popular during the period after the Spanish-American War (1898) and named for U.S. Navy hero Admiral George Dewey (1837-1917).

digger. Term for a soldier. First applied to Australian Expeditionary Forces during World War I.

doughboy. The term used for American soldiers in Europe during World War I.

DMZ. Demilitarized zone.

EGA. Eagle, Globe, and Anchor. The device worn on the hat and collars of a Marine uniform.

E. Pluribus Unum. From many one.

escutcheon. A diamond-, shield-, or oval-shaped plate on the wrist of a rifle, pistol, knife, or sword. The term is sometimes used to denote the shield on insignia.

flat cap. Sometimes referred to as Donald Duck hat. A tallied cap used by the navies of the world during the 19th and early-20th centuries.

gabardine. A blended fabric used by the military to make uniforms.

G.A.R. Grand Army of the Republic. Society for Union troop veterans of the Civil War.

HBT. Herringbone twill. Type of fabric used in abundance during World War II and in the Korean War. Known for its durability.

H.M.S. His/Her Majesty's Ship.

Hussar. Type of German Cavalry.

kindersabel. German for child's (*kinder*) sabre (*sabel*).

Kriegsmarine. German Navy.

MACV. Military Assistance Command Vietnam. Pronounced *Mac-V.* It was headquarters to General William Westmoreland and a clearinghouse for all command during the Vietnam Conflict.

Mameluke. Modeled after the scimitar (sword), it is a highly regarded symbol of the United States Marine Corps Officers Corps. Its brass diamond-shaped crossguard, ivory slab grips, and pierced pommel are its distinctive characteristics.

MIA. Missing in action.

militia. A sometimes elite organization of volunteers involved in military training at a local level. Militias were incorporated into active service in the event of a state or national emergency.

Montana Peak hat. A campaign hat adopted by the U.S. Army from 1911 to 1940. It continues to be used by present-day Marines.

NCO. Non-commissioned officer.

NOS. New old stock.

OG. Olive green. Denotes a fabric color; i.e., OG-107 is a specific color variant.

OD. Olive-drab. Denotes the color of uniform fabric.

plume socket. The metal socket used to hold a feather or horsehair plume on the top of a military hat.

OS cap. Overseas cap.

powder monkey. Slang term used for boys serving in gun batteries of ships. They brought up the black powder to those loading gun barrels.

puttees. Leg wrappings or coverings worn by Army troops prior to and during World War I.

quatrefoil. Decoration on the sleeve of a military jacket.

RAF. Royal Air Force (England).

RCAF. Royal Canadian Air Force.

sabertash. A decorative bag similar in size to a cartridge box and worn suspended by a shoulder belt across the chest. The children's version was usually just a small plate of brass with a decorative motif stamped in.

Sam Browne. A dress belt used by officers. "Sam" stands for Uncle Sam issue and "Browne" denotes that it was made of brown leather.

tintype. Images produced on thin sheets of iron painted with Japan varnish. This process was used from the late 1850s until around 1930.

tombeau. The cloverleaf design on a Zouave jacket.

UCV. United Confederate Veterans. Society for Confederate veterans of the Civil War.

WAAC. Women's Auxiliary Army Corps, which became WAC on September 30, 1943.

WAC. Women's Army Corps.

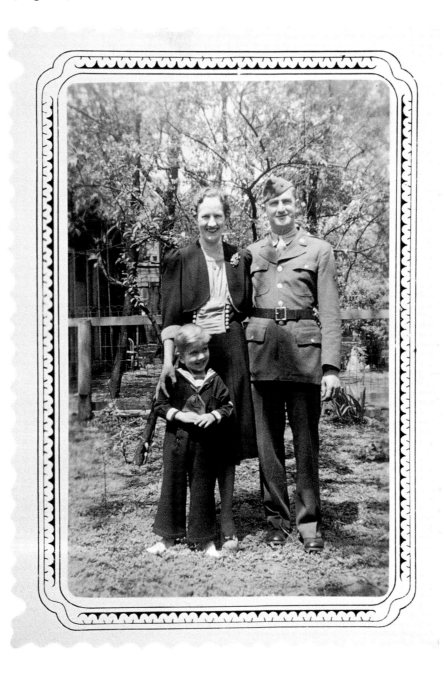

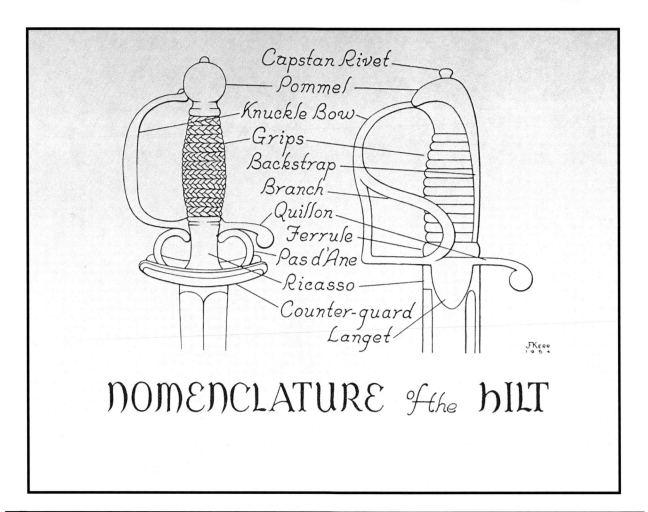

NOMENCLATURE of the HILT

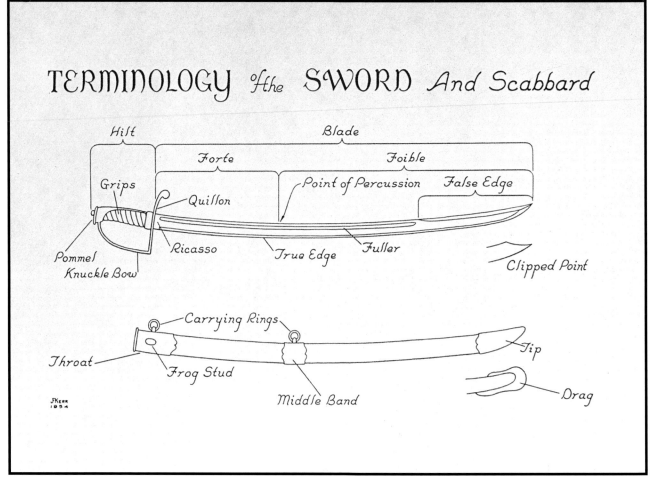

TERMINOLOGY of the SWORD And Scabbard

Detailed Buying Guide

Sooner or later all collectors and dealers ask one distinctive question that brings them together or sets them apart: "What is it worth?"

Finding an object at a yard sale for one dollar and selling it for one hundred dollars does not determine the value. Truth be known, in most cases, nothing could be further from the truth. In the case of this book, as of the first printing, no other interpretations have previously been written on this particular collecting genre. Our only point of reference thus far has been the occasional example in references on American Home Front items, and a small pocket of European collectors whose main interest is based on the emphasis of correctness to the adult uniform counterparts. Note: These prices only reflect what we have seen similar items bought and sold for in the past.

In the case of American children's costumes and equipage we see a 180-degree turnabout. Many of the items you have seen in this reference are homemade, and as such, possess uniqueness and cleverness of design.

In short, rarity almost never determines price. Historical value, condition, materials, visual impact, desire, and bargaining skills should ultimately determine the prices an individual collector pays. During the course of collecting material for this book, I was offered many items at prices that I would consider too high. However, I quickly learned that sometimes all it takes is a gracious "no thank you" to bring the price down significantly. Conversely, I have turned down many items at prices that don't seem so high now, and I kick myself for being so stubborn. Live and learn.

While evaluating the wide range in prices listed here, bear in mind travel expenses, time, and the knowledge it requires to sort through the many oysters to find "the pearl." Values follow trends, which spike up and down in all phases of the collectibles market. Another factor to consider when shopping for collectibles is regional interest. For example, Civil War collectibles are valued somewhat higher in the southern and northeastern regions of this country where they enjoy a broader following. Outside the US where American collectibles are

scarcer, prices may be significantly higher. Taking extra time to learn as much as you can about your particular collecting interest and staying firmly within the guidelines you set for yourself will ultimately save you time, money, and a lot of heartache. My husband, Steve, has told me more times than I can recall, "You buy your education in this business." I have learned the hard way that *you buy what you want because you like it*, not because you made yourself believe it's a wise investment. With that in mind, understand that the following information in this buying guide is just that, "a guide."

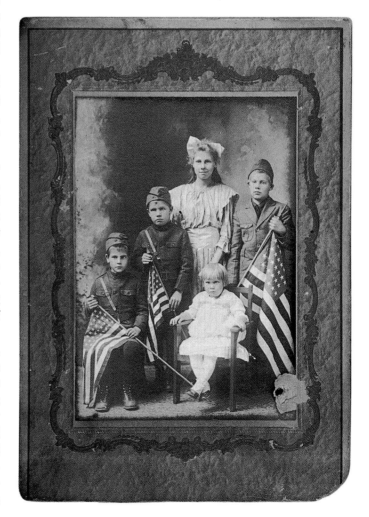

Images

When purchasing pre-1900 photographic images from this genre, try to stay within the bounds of the collecting guidelines you have set. Though interesting, many images of boys in school or cadet uniforms are confused with child fantasy soldiers as seen in this book. Conversely, children dressed in regular "fashion of the day" (especially the Civil War era) are commonly mistaken for "children in uniform." Elements within the image are critical to determining value and may be overlooked on a casual first glance.

As the 20th century dawned, photographers were very productive, and eager families made the journey to have photographs taken in many settings. For children during this time, we see a trend in the number of both girls and boys dressed in highly stylized Navy attire, then, as war becomes a certainty in Europe, we see a sudden shift to accurate Army-style uniforms on boys. Those who specifically collect images know that the photographic record left behind from this period is staggering, but not fully explored. While, at present, photos of children in military apparel from this time frame may seem rare, my personal experience dictates that they are actually quite common.

During the years of World War II, photography became available for home use and many families owned their own cameras, so again we see a shift in format from formal studio settings to less formal home settings and simple unmounted snapshots.

Photographic images come in several types, sizes, and formats. For a definition of formats, see the glossary. Below are pricing guidelines for an image of a child in an American fantasy uniform with a single accoutrement; i.e. a drum, flag, toy or a sword, gun etc. Multiple accoutrements, elaborate detail, specific backmarks (regional interest), or, in the example of hard images, cased images framed by a stamped brass mat will increase value accordingly.

Daguerreotype	$400-600+
Ambrotype	$300-500+
Tintype	$75-200
CDV Carte de Viste	$35-75
Albumen	$15-50
Cabinet Card	$5-20
Stereo View Card	$3-10
Paper Photograph/Postcard	
WWI:	$2-25
WWII:	$1-15
Korea:	$1-5
Vietnam:	$3-8

After the turn of the 20th century, photography became more standardized, and was simplified to unmounted paper images; however, one can still encounter tintype photography into the early 1920s.

Earlier photography will obviously have increased value. When shopping for pre-1870 images it is important to remember condition is everything and damage significantly reduces value, regardless of content. Also, don't be surprised if large-format photography prices from all periods are somewhat higher.

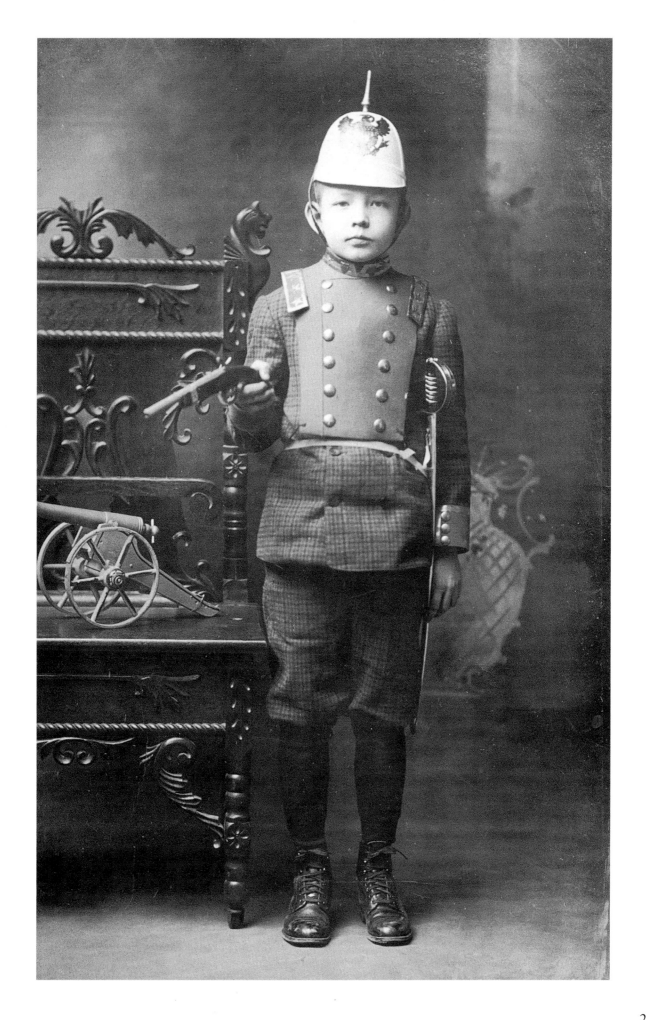

Swords

Swords have always carried a place of prominence among collectors, and their interest remains quite appealing. Given these facts, children's swords are usually found in one of four types. (For sword nomenclature and terminology see page 208.) Though there are many subcategories of the four types described here, this should give the reader a basic outline of what is available in the collecting market.

Type 1. Made from the exact materials and patterns of their adult counterpart. These scaled-down versions exhibit exacting detail in all respects, including engraved or etched blades, the use of silver and gold gilt finishes, and fullered blades. Many times when one encounters a sword of this quality, it can be surmised it was given or presented to the son of an important military or political figure.

Type 2. Swords that were commercially manufactured as adult swords, which have been, for whatever reason, cut down for use by a child or adolescent boy. These original swords, (i.e. Cadet, Musician, NCO, and others) have been altered by cutting down the blade and scabbard and were mostly used by military schools and cadets. As there were hundreds of military schools and academies around the country prior to the turn of the 20th century, it is likely that when one encounters a sword of this quality, one can presume it was for this purpose. Rarely were swords of this type just handed over to a young boy to play with in the backyard. Though they may appear to be relatively harmless, they are formidable weapons and should be respected as such. Since swords of this type are not true children's swords, it is the opinion of the author that this type does not fit into the collecting genre represented in this book.

Type 3. Commercially manufactured child's swords ranging from variations of American or European adult styles to pure fantasy swords. Materials for swords of this type include plated, low-grade metal, tin, wood, leather, or even the occasional genuine sharkskin grip. Specimens from this type rarely have a cutting edge or fullered blade. The tips are usually (but not always) blunt or rounded, offering some protection from injury. Though these were readily available until around the beginning of World War II, many could not stand up to the abuses, and they have not survived in vast numbers. Most, as a rule, will display the inherent problems of bent blades, dented or missing scabbards, missing parts, or broken or loose hilts.

Type 4. Swords made at home or in small metal or wood shops. In the case of this type, you may find a sword which was made up for a child's toy or as a prop. Materials will vary from wood to whatever was available or on-hand; the degree of workmanship is generally somewhat poor; however, swords of this type were made in large numbers for boys during World War II because of restrictions on vital materials. Though not highly prized monetarily, these swords display one of the author's favorite aspects of children's military-style accoutrements, the true fantasy of soldiering.

Note: During World War II, "scrap drives" claimed many swords, adult and child's alike. A US Government poster campaign stating "Give a Knife, Save a Life" pressed into service many unlikely edged weapons and cutting instruments. Surplus and collected adult sword blades and knives were remanufactured into fighting or "combat" knives that went to American servicemen overseas. Even children were encouraged to turn in a variety of metal toys (including swords) to aid the war effort. Later, during the Korean and Vietnam eras, swords became less prominent in boys' fantasy military play, and were largely replaced with wood or plastic automatic-style guns. Most toy swords seen during this time were made from mold-injected plastic and with few exceptions do not reflect the pre-1900 military-style swords used in America and abroad.

Type 1 Pre-Civil War-1890	$150-500+
Type 2	$100-350+
Type 3	$35-150
Type 4	$25-45

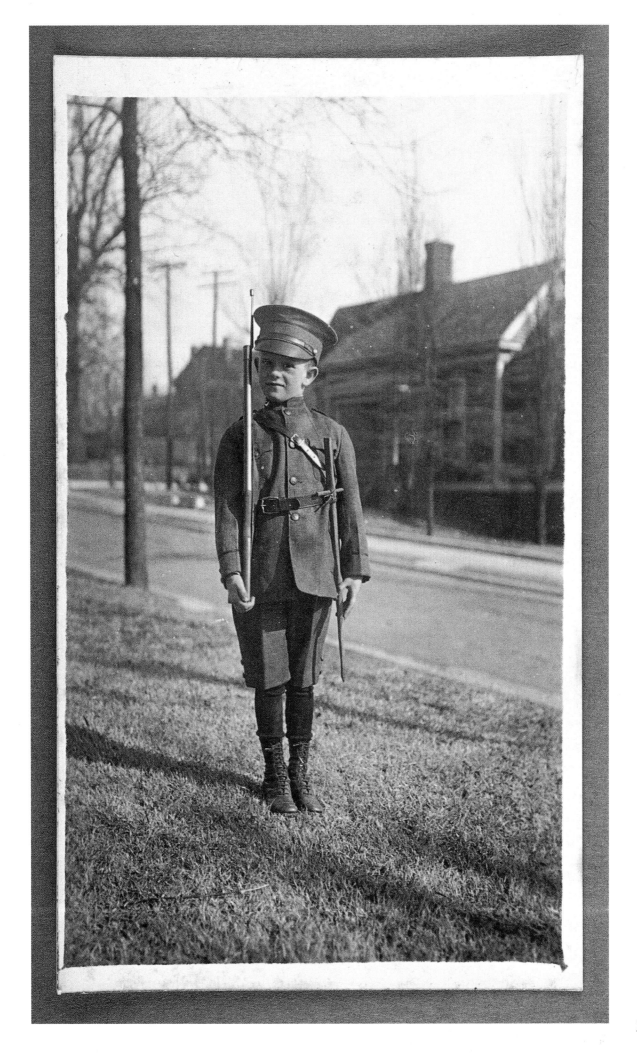

Drums

Drums made for children from the 1850 through the Civil War are, by and large, scaled-down versions of adult military-style drums. Though smaller in all dimensions they are constructed of wood with skin-heads mounted with roped wooden rims. Many have painted patriotic themes such as shields, flags, and eagles. Condition varies greatly on drums from this time period, and most seem to need some degree of repair. This is not uncommon, but if repaired incorrectly, the value of the drum is reduced significantly.

Caution should be used when considering the purchase of an early drum. As stated previously, because of the number of military schools and academies during the latter half of the 19th century, scaled-down drums are not always toys. Professionally made, scaled-down drums may be a remnant of the schools, and would not be included in the fantasy soldier category.

Having had the opportunity to visit Noble & Cooley & Company, one of the oldest drum manufacturers in the US, and viewing their large collection from many eras, I observed that they maintain the notion of "keep it simple" when it comes to toy drums. After the 1890s manufacturing techniques switched from wood and rope to metal embossed bodies, rims, and springs. Patriotic emblems, soldiers, flags, cannons, ships, and more were screen-painted on in exacting detail. Tin and heavy-gauge paper heads replaced skin-heads.

Later, some manufacturers utilized "tin-can manufacturing for toy drums," producing an empty one-piece drum, which was in fact a large painted tin can. Holes were punched through the rim to accommodate string slings.

As World War II restrictions were placed on toy manufacturers, construction from stamped, heavy-gauge cardboard became necessary for the duration of the war. But by the end of the war, drum prominence in boys' war play had receded into obscurity. No longer did boys dream of being a brave drummer marching toward the front.

Note: Drum prices at the high side should be "excellent +" condition. Price guidelines for the below drums would include examples of toy drums manufactured for play, and not the scaled-down drums used by boys at military schools or academies.

Drum- Complete 1850-1865	$200-350+
With Artwork	$400-600
Drum Complete 1865-1895	$75-200
Tin Drum 1895-1940	$ 35-150
WWII Paper drum-Excellent	$50-75

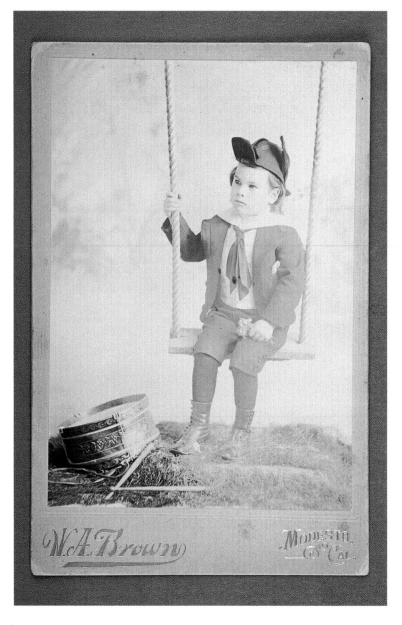

Headgear

Realistic military-style hats have always been an important part of a child's fantasy of soldiering. For a child with a good imagination a military-style hat can be the centerpiece of a pretend uniform. As military headgear has evolved and changed through the history of this country, so has children's toy military headgear. During the Civil War, we see many children donning small kepis with play insignia sewn on. Later, photographic evidence supports that toy helmets replicating 1872 and 1881 patterns were worn by children of means while fighting the "Indians" in their backyards.

Once again when considering the purchase of a pre-1900 kepi for a collection, remember that kepis in several designs were used by the military of this country for over 40 years. Some people mistakenly identify all kepis as "Civil War" period headgear. For a new collector in this field, a study of 19th-century military headgear will prove profitable in several respects. Peaks, slopes, and brim styles on kepi headgear evolved during the period of its use by the military. Also, because kepis were used by military schools and academies during this period, it is worth familiarizing yourself with the styles and insignias used by these institutions so you are not purchasing a school cap.

As America entered World War I, we see the beginnings of widespread use of "steel pot" helmets. During the 1930s MARX Toy Company was faithful in answering the cry of the armies of boys who wanted realistic steel helmets to fight the Germans in the woods. These helmets occasionally can still be found with the "shock-proof pad" that was fastened to the inside top of the helmet to avoid injury while running. This pad was a formed disk of pressed fiber and pop-riveted to the inside center of the top of the helmet. A string, cord, or elastic band fastened to the rim held the helmets in place. Child versions of this "doughboy" helmet were popular right up to the World War II restrictions on vital materials. A pressed fiberboard helmet replaced the steel helmets for the duration of that war. In the 1950s we see steel helmets replaced with plastic helmets with netting in the World War II style.

Campaign and Overseas-style hats are also important to fantasy soldiering. During World War II children could buy surplus and small-size World War I OS caps. Those made specifically for children were manufactured and available in toy stores and five-and-dimes. Bond and scrap drives rewarded the industrious child with a "stamped" OS cap as shown in Chapter 8. During the Vietnam era, toy "Boonie" hats were popular with boys playing war.

Of all the headgear I have collected, the flying helmets are among my favorites. Leather helmets of varying quality have made their way to my collection, and I love all of them. The romance of the aviator has never waned in military and civilian life in America. Toy goggles fall into the category with flying helmets. Some flying helmets were manufactured with goggles attached; some came with them unattached, and some goggles

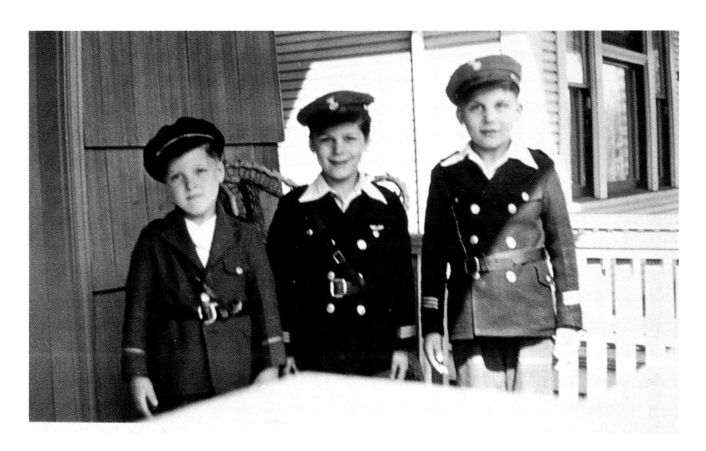

were sold separately. Once the war was over and we were sitting on the bubble of the jet-age, the leather-flying helmet became a casualty of aviation technology. Fortunately, in its many forms it maintains a place as a beloved memory for the many people whose childhood intersected with the years leading up to and during World War II. My father, who was a child during World War II growing up in Los Angeles, fondly remembers the desire to own a real flying helmet. My grandmother, being a practical woman, refused to buy anything that even remotely resembled a fleece-lined snow hat, claiming it was far too warm to wear such a thing.

For further details of types of flying helmets, see Chapter 8.

Below prices are for headgear in excellent + to very good condition.

Child's Kepi	
1861-1865	$400-600+
1865-1890	$150-275+
19th Century	
1872 & 1881 Pattern	
helmets	$50-175
Overseas Cap	
WWI	$5-20
WWII	$5-30

Navy Flat Cap	
(Donald Duck Hat)	$5-25
Unique specimens featuring	
Cap-tallies from	
Historically Significant	
ships	$20-50
Helmet- Steel	$15-50
Squadron Marked/	
MARX (Condition)	$35-50
Helmet-WWII Fiberboard	
/Jr. Commando	$35-75
Helmet- Plastic	$5-15
Flying Helmet	
Leather/Lined	$15-40
Leather/Unlined	$20-50
Adult Helmet Modified	
for Child Use	$25-75
Visor Cap	$10-30
Unusual Visor Cap	$20-35
Higher Quality w/ Military	
Correctness & Deluxe	
Trimmings	$20-65
Steve Canyon Flying	
Helmet (In Box)	$35-75

Uniforms

Uniforms and stylized costumes are a difficult area to cover completely. Prior to World War I the majority were made at home or privately tailored. During World War I, commercial manufacturers saw the opportunity to capitalize on the patriotic home-front trend and began offering "boxed costume uniforms" for boys through catalog sales. These early styles replicated not only service uniforms, such as "doughboys," but also cadet uniforms. Later on, as the aviation trend grew in popularity, aviator costumes came center stage, offering multi-piece, boxed costumes that include headgear, goggles, and Sam Browne belts. In the World War II years, girls came into the act dressed as WACs and WAVEs, and boys wanted to dress like Navy lieutenants and Air Force captains like they saw in the movies.

Boxed costumes from about the late 1930s forward are characterized by many elements, including inexpensive fabrics and buttons, pot-metal insignia, and plastic headbands in the hats. Many styles had elastic waistband in the trousers, dispensing with the expense of button/zipper flies.

A slightly higher quality of ready-to-wear outfit was also popular during World War II, which utilized a higher quality of fabrics, buttons, and fly closures. Hats included in this type of stylized uniform are usually multi-piece construction "crusher"-style caps. Styles most often seen from this category include khaki Air Force styles and Navy sailor suits. Because of the low prices on these costumes, high sentiment, many working moms, and the willingness of children to wear them, we see few homemade costumes from this era. Professional tailor-made uniforms are far more common, especially for those of significant means.

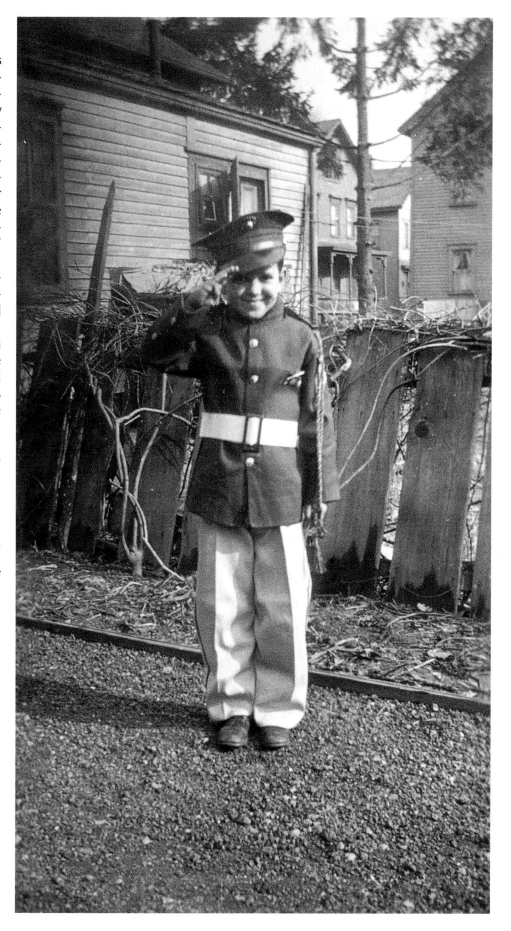

Costumes found in their original boxes will obviously command higher prices. Boxes that display elaborate box art can be expected to bring higher prices still.

The trend of "officer" costumes faded as the Vietnam era began, and we see a shift back to enlisted-style costumes such as Marine Rangers and Green Berets. The other area of Vietnam collectibles is "in-country-made" items. This is a completely different category since the majority of the value will sit within the insignia, fabric, styles, and patterns themselves. Opportunities to purchase child-size uniforms in Saigon and other areas where US personnel were stationed were a common occurrence during the war. Some of the best insignia and camo material was available and created some very impressive children's uniforms. The best tailor shops could create a uniform with direct-embroidered insignia, which was identical to adult counterparts. This is a fascinating area for collecting; however, it is already an established market with Vietnam collectors, so be prepared to do your homework on insignia, fabrics, and patterns. As children's pieces might expect to bring slightly lower prices than adult uniforms, understand that because of the lack of certain patterns, children's uniforms could easily wind up as a beret or hat to be funneled back into the adult Vietnam collectors' market. For a visual identification of the many patterns and peripheral tour jackets and party suits, see Chapter 10.

Handmade uniforms and stylized costumes can probably be closely matched in prices to vintage clothing. Remember, because of high trends in all phases of patriotism during World War II, uniform styles from that era should not be considered rare. Also because this is the first book of its kind, at the time of the first printing, children's military and patriotic collectibles are young markets. As more people become interested in these collecting genre, there is no telling the volume of material that may turn up. As it has been observed in many other areas of collecting, when an interest is generated and new supplies become available the prices will be affected. When considering the purchase of a child's uniform or stylized costume, ask yourself if it contains more elements that are geared toward a child's fantasy or if the item contains too many adult insignia and patch elements. Articles loaded with adult insignia and patches are easy to produce for a hungry market and may not be a period-made.

The following prices are for generalized commercially manufactured uniforms. High-end prices are for complete uniforms in excellent to very good condition. A premium can be added for uniqueness, visual appeal, boxed condition, and handmade or professionally tailored one-of-a-kind items. The descriptions below are what the author considers to be the most commonly found items a collector would encounter at a swap meet, flea market or antique mall/shop.

World War I

Boxed Uniform/ In Box	$150-300
Common Army or Navy	$35-50
Navy Peacoat w/Hat	$25-45

World War II

Boxed Uniform for boys, girl WAC, WAVE COMMANDO, 5-Star General, etc.	$50-150
Special Uniforms with Extra Correct Insignia, Visor Hats, Sam Browne Belts, Waist Belt, Purse, and Other Accessories	$50-150

Korea/Vietnam

Special Service Uniforms, i.e. USMC Green Beret, Special Forces Ranger, Astronaut	$65-200
Vietnam In-Country-Made Uniforms, Shirts, Tour Jackets, Party Suits, etc.	$35-200

Miscellaneous

While gathering material for this book, I had more fun with the items in this category than I did any other. It is amazing to me what corporate America believes is patriotic. Commercially manufactured home-front items range from downright cool to unbelievably tacky.

You may discover that insignia are the toughest to buy in this category. Once again, your best opportunities to buy insignia made and designed especially for children will be in items from the World War II period. Unlike any other time before, the media, via radio and Hollywood, heavily influenced children. With so much going on, children became very sophisticated very quickly, and the demand for more realistic military play toys was high.

Cereal and other foodstuff premiums will be a tremendous source for insignia. Many of the items you saw in Chapter 8, including a steel pot helmet, wings, iron-on and leather squadron patches, are premiums. Premiums are awards for mailing in labels from products, then waiting impatiently for the six to eight weeks it took to get the items back. Premiums were a huge market for children of the radio age, and almost all children's radio-show characters had a story line that included the war at one point or another.

Boots are another item that fall in this category. As I mentioned in Chapter 8, what may look like an Army style boot today was actually just a shoe for boys back then. Two buckle boots had a wide variety of stamped flaps in the military motif, and I find new ones all the time.

The high-side prices below would represent items in Excellent to Very Good condition.

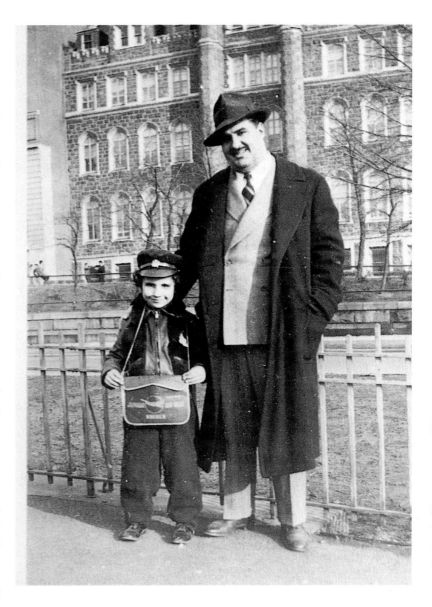

Leather Items

Two Buckle Boots w/	
Military Motif Stamp	$20-65
Sam Browne Leather Belt	$5-20
Sam Brown Belt w/Holster	$15-50
MacArthur Holster & Gun	$20-70
AF/USMC/Army	
Holster & Gun	$15-50

Canteens

Civil War	$65-125
1865-1900	$35-100
WWII	$5-25
Korea/Vietnam (mess	
kits also)	$5-15
Pre-WWII Period	
Army/AF Backpack/	
Book Bag	$35-75

Insignia

Jr. Pilot, Paratrooper,	
Bombardier etc. (painted	
pot metal)	$10-25
Jr. Flight Nurse	$15-25
Jr. Crackerjack Pilot	$50-75
American Boy Outfit on	
Card	$15-35
Victory Tattoos On	
Card- Complete	$15-25
Leatherette Squadron	
Patch-Premium (each)	$3-7

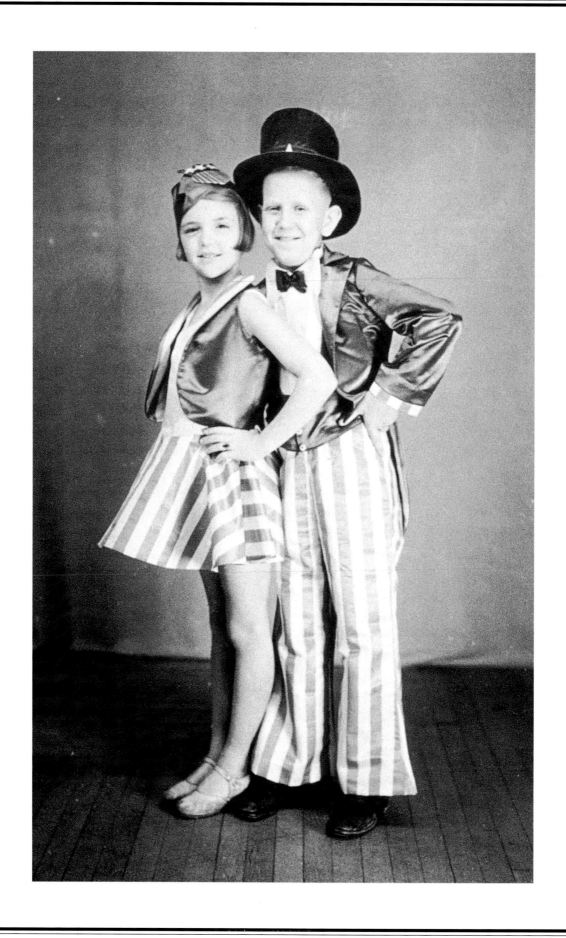

Bibliography

Albert, Alphaeus H. *Record of American Uniform and Historical Buttons – Bicentennial Edition*. Hightown, New Jersey: Albert, 1977.

Bunley, J.W. *Military & Naval Recognition Book* New York, New York: Van Nostrand Company Inc., 1942.

Caba, G. Craig. *United States Military Drums 1845-1865: A Pictorial Survey*. Harrisburg, Pennsylvania: Civil War Antiquities and Americana, 1977.

Campbell, J. Duncan. *Aviation Badges and Insignia of the United States Army 1913-1946*. Harrisburg, Pennsylvania: Triangle Press, 1977.

French Navy Web site. http: // www.<marine.national.sirpa.<mer @ wandoo.fr

Howell, Edgar M. *United States Army Headgear 1855-1902*. Fredricksburg, Virginia: North South Press, 1986.

Kerkis, Sydney C. *Plates and Buckles of the American Military: 1795-1874*. Stone Mountain, Georgia: Stone Mountain Press, 1986.

Langellier, John P. *Army Blue: The Uniforms of Uncle Sam's Regulars 1848-1873*. Atglen, Pennsylvania: Schiffer Military History, 1998.

Lewis, Kenneth. *Doughboy to GI Army Clothing and Equipment 1900-1945* West Midland, England: Norman D. Landing Publishing, 1993.

Matthews, Jack. *Toys Go To War* Pictorial Histories Publishing Company Inc., Missoula, Montana 1994

Mace, O. Henry. *Collector's Guide to Early Photographs*. Radnor, Pennsylvania: Wallace-Homestead Book Co., 1990.

McAfee, Michael J. *Zouaves: The First and the Bravest*. Gettysburg, Pennsylvania: Thomas Publications, 1991.

McCombs, Don and Fred L. Worth. *World War II: Super Facts*. New York: Warner Publishing, 1983.

McNeil, Alex. *Total Television: The Comprehensive Guide to Programming From 1948 to the Present*. New York: Penguin Books, 1996.

Mowbray, E. Andrew and Stuart C. Mowbray. "The Young Cavaliers," *Man at Arms Magazine*, Lincoln, Rhode Island, 1997.

Moore, Warren. *Weapons of the American Revolution and Accoutrements*. New York: Promontory Press, 1967.

Neuman, George C. *Swords & Blades of the American Revolution* Harrisburg, Pennsylvania: Stackpole Books, 1973.

O'Donnell, Michael J. and Duncan Campbell. *American Military Belt Plates 1996*. Alexandria, Virginia: O'Donnell Publishing, 1996.

Peterson, Harold L. *The American Sword 1775-1945, Revised Edition*. Philadelphia, Pennsylvania: Ray Riling Arms Books Co., 1965.

Philips, Stanley S. *Civil War Corps Badges and Other Related Awards, Badges, Medals of the Period*. Langham, Maryland: Stanley S. Philips, 1982.

Prisoner-of-war information: http://www.scopesys.com/powmia/.

Todd, Fredrick P. *American Military Equipage 1851-1872*. Providence, Rhode Island: Mowbray Company-Publishers, 1978.

Williams, Col. Dion. *Army and Navy Uniforms and Insignia*. New York: Fredrick A. Stones, 1918.

Zipper information: http://www.kusm.montana.edu/wordsmith/words/0010.html and http://www.mining.com.

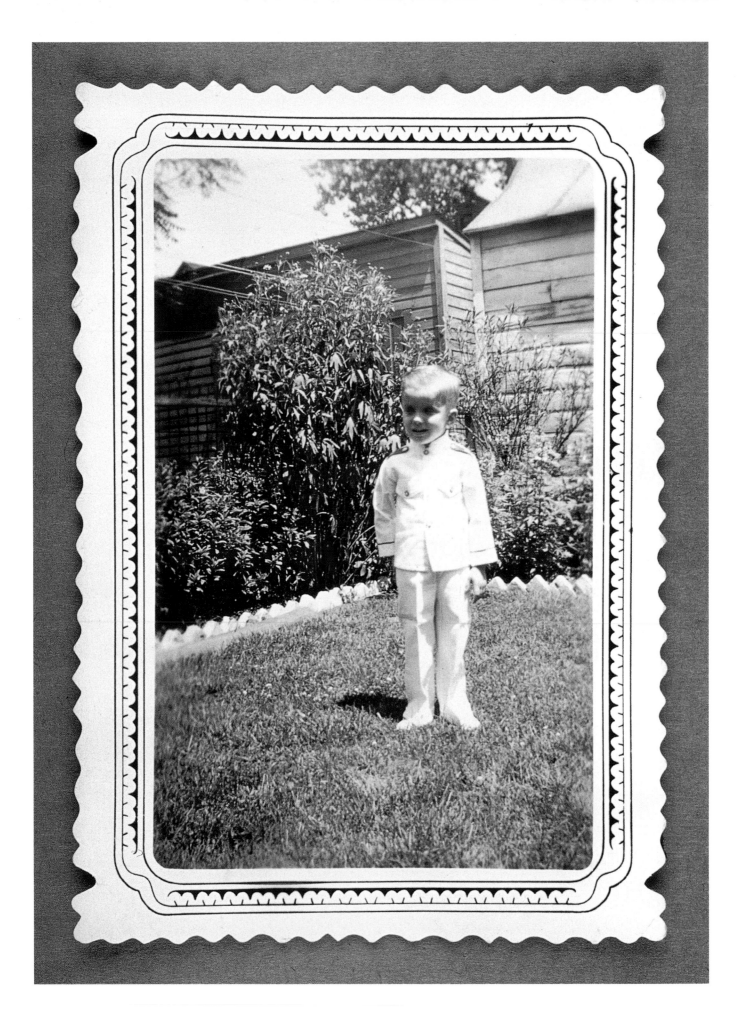

Author's Note

The best lessons of history come about when they make a connection to our individual lives. For myself the true spirit of patriotism was demonstrated in a tangible way on countless occasions during my childhood, which began and ended parallel to the years of American involvement in Southeast Asia.

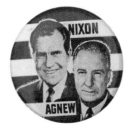

I recall with utter joy when I shared with my classmates at Show-n-Tell the story of how Mom chased down and recaptured an American flag from a group of teenagers who stole it from a local polling place. At breakneck speed, she raced her VW Bug through the neighborhood, until she cornered them, scolded them, and without a word to anyone, replaced it in its proper place before going back to the school gymnasium to vote. I learned two important life lessons that day: don't mess with the American flag and don't mess with Mom.

My third-grade teacher, a Hawaiian woman of Japanese descent, took it upon herself to make sure every child who passed through her classroom knew and understood the meaning of every word of the Pledge of Allegiance. A precious gift.

I also recall the day my father came home with a POW/MIA bracelet. Once a week he would take it off and polish the copper band, then slip it back on his wrist, a commitment to remember that went on for years until March 4, 1973, when I saw him cry as he removed it for the last time. We watched from our living room with full hearts as Capt. Harold Johnson, a POW since April 30, 1967, stepped off the C-141 at Clarks AFB in the Philippines and back to freedom.

Fond memories of my mother and I baking cookies for GIs during Thanksgiving vacation hold special meaning. Each cookie was wrapped and nestled down into fresh popcorn inside the huge film canisters my dad would bring home from the studios in Burbank. The canisters were sealed, addressed to men who were total strangers to our family, and then mailed off to Vietnam. As a child, I often wondered if the cookies my mother and I had baked with so much care ever reached or gave comfort to any of the faces I saw nightly on the evening news.

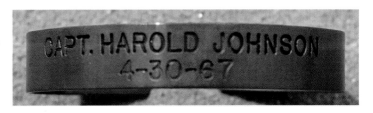

What I tried to share within these pages are the memories and patriotic pride of children from their point of view. If you have photos, stories, or items you would like to share for future editions of *Wee Warriors & Playtime Patriots*, please contact me through Schiffer Books, or at the website below.

If this or any other Schiffer Military History publication has impressed or inspired you and you would like to donate one or more to a public or school library at institutional pricing, please contact Schiffer Books at 610-593-1777 for a catalog of titles

Plant the seed of patriotism in a child's heart.

Visit us at www.playtimepatriots.com .

-NG

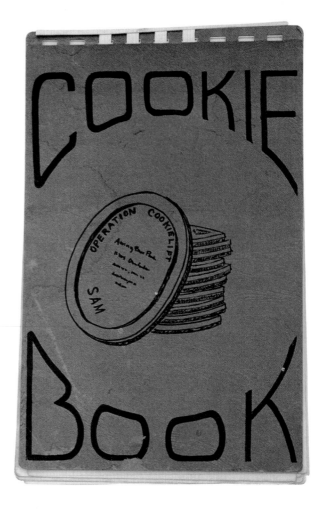

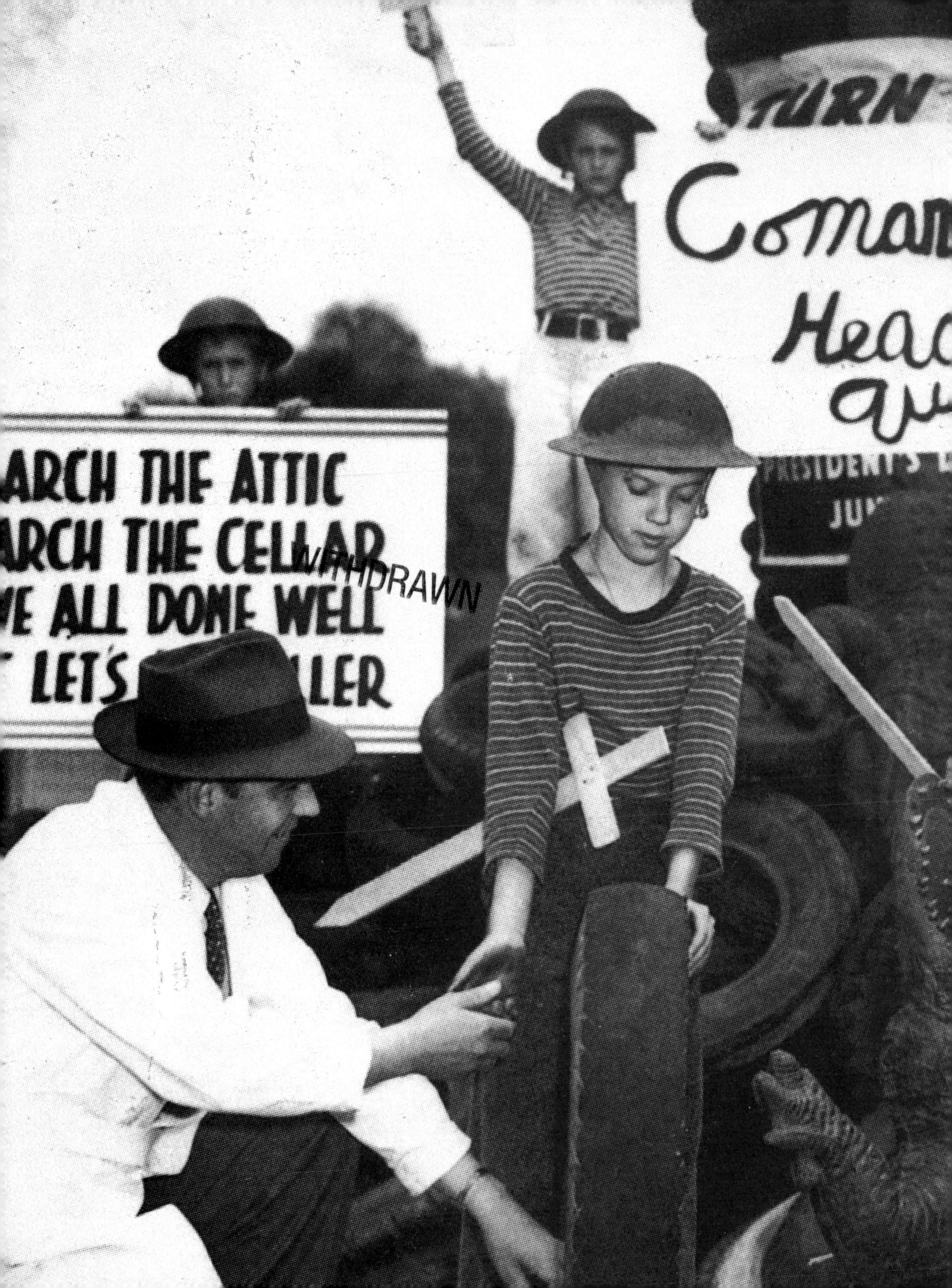
ARCH THE ATTIC
ARCH THE CELLAR
E ALL DONE WELL
LET'S LLER
TURN